GUIDE TO
RESTAURANT
FOOD
JOSEPH C. PISCATELLA

Workman Publishing, New York

**Library of Congress
Cataloging-in-Publication Data**

Piscatella, Joseph C.
    The fat-gram guide to restaurant food.
       p.   cm.
    ISBN 0-7611-0950-1 (alk. paper)
    1. Restaurants—United States—
Guidebooks.   2. Food—Fat content.
3. Low-fat diet.   I. Title.
TX907.2.P57   1998
647.9573—dc21   97-45608
                                CIP

Workman books are available at special discount when purchased in bulk for special sales promotions as well as fund-raising or educational use. Special book excerpts or editions can also be created to specification. For details, contact the Special Sales Director at the address below.

Workman Publishing Company, Inc.
708 Broadway
New York, 10003

First printing February 1998
Manufactured in the United States
10 9 8 7 6 5 4 3 2 1

CONTENTS

The information in this book should not be construed as medical advice or instruction. Always consult your physician or other appropriate health professionals before making dietary changes.

INTRODUCTION

C hances are, the reason you've picked up this book is that you'd like to cut the fat in your diet in order to lose weight and/or reduce cholesterol. Perhaps you're already cooking with less fat—using non-stick pans and cooking sprays, for example. And you might be doing a better job in grocery stores of reading food labels for nutrition information. But if you're like most people, you're still having difficulty in determining the fat content of restaurant foods.

The problem for consumers is that restaurant foods lack nutrition labels, so most of us have only a general idea of their fat content. Oh, we know that these foods tend to be richer in fat. It's no secret that restaurant meals often contain liberal amounts of butter, oil, cream, lard, mayonnaise, meat drippings, fatty meat, cheese and cheese sauce. In addition, restaurants often fry or deep-fry, which can increase the fat content of their food. And finally, many restaurants offer huge portions, so fat intake is increased simply by the amount of food eaten.

But we don't always recognize which restaurant foods are fat or how fat they are. For instance, we might identify a McDonald's Big Mac as a high-fat food (although we probably don't know it has 31 grams of fat). We don't have a clue, however, that two packets of McDonald's Ranch Salad Dressing actually has more fat— 42 grams! Or that an average order of cheese nachos—about 55 grams of fat—is the same as eating about three Burger King cheeseburgers.

Such confusion over fat content, coupled with the trend toward eating out more often, has contributed greatly to America's weight problem. It's no coincidence that as we've come to rely more on restaurant foods, our weight has gone up. It's estimated that during the past five years restaurant meals have risen to half of all meals consumed in the U.S. (When Americans are asked "What are you making for dinner?" the answer is often "Reservations.") But over this same five-year period, the average American has gained eight pounds.

Reducing dietary fat is an indispensable key to weight loss and cholesterol reduction. But you can't cut fat if you don't know where it is. So, you have two options regarding restaurant foods. You can give them up altogether, which isn't very realistic. Or you can make smarter choices about the restaurant foods you order. This is where a restaurant fat-gram counter will help. With over 3,500 sit-down and fast-food items listed, this book is a comprehensive guide to the fat content of restaurant foods. It is a tool to help you make better food decisions.

DIETARY FAT: A PROPER PERSPECTIVE

Everyone today seems to be trying to avoid dietary fat. But fat often takes a bad rap. The truth is that in itself, there is nothing wrong with dietary fat. It makes food taste better, it helps to distribute flavors throughout the mouth and keeps them there longer, and it provides texture. Fat also adds moisture to food, causing it literally to "melt in your mouth." And because you digest it slowly, it provides an enjoyable feeling of satisfaction after a meal. In addition, it promotes good health by providing essential fatty acids and transporting vitamins A, D, E and K.

Excessive dietary fat, however, is a health concern. A high-fat diet is linked to elevated cholesterol, heart disease, stroke, certain cancers, diabetes, high blood pressure, gallbladder disease, osteoarthritis and the nation's leading ailment—obesity. The connection between diet and health/appearance is well documented and is the reason most Americans are so interested in reducing fat. Organizations such as the American Heart Association and the National Cancer Institute recommend eating a diet with less than 30% of calories from fat.

Given this concern, there's a widespread popular belief that the American diet has become substantially leaner in the last few years. "Not so," says Bonnie Liebman, a registered dietitian at the Center for Science in the Public Interest. "Today we get about 34% of calories from fat, so it appears that we're eating less than in the late 1970s, when fat constituted over 40% of calories. But fat reduction is a myth. What we're eating today is not a lower-fat diet. *It's a higher-calorie diet.* We are actually eating slightly more fat today than in 1991, but we're taking in a lot more calories. So the percentage looks better, but the actual amount of fat has not fallen. And that's why we're not losing weight. The recommendation to cut back on fat means just that: Eat less fat. If these numbers reflect what people are eating, we're in trouble."

The truth is that fatty foods, particularly restaurant foods like cheeseburgers, French fries, fried chicken, prime rib and Caesar salad, continue to be at the center of the American diet. Such foods are largely responsible for the fact that the average American eats between 800 and 1,000 calories every day as fat, or about the equivalent of one full stick of butter. As one doctor put it, "This is a nation that discusses its weight problems over Danish pastry!"

Is it possible, then, to live a modern lifestyle and still trim fat from restaurant foods? The answer is yes. Here's how you do it.

ESTABLISH YOUR FAT BUDGET

The first thing you should do is establish your personal fat budget, which will answer this fundamental question: "How much fat can I eat today and still be on a lean, healthy diet?" By determining the maximum amount of fat you can eat, your budget becomes a guideline for the day and a standard against which to measure your food choices. After all, it doesn't make much sense to know how much fat comes in a tuna sandwich if you don't know how that amount fits into your daily fat budget.

A personal fat budget should be just that—personal. Each person and each lifestyle is different. An "average" figure for all men or all women may not reflect the best budget for you. You can calculate your own fat budget in three simple steps.

STEP 1: DETERMINE YOUR IDEAL WEIGHT

An individual's scale weight is less important than what makes up that weight—how much is lean muscle and bone, and how much is fat. Suppose two people each weigh 100 pounds on a scale. But if one is 90 pounds of muscle and 10 pounds of fat, while the other is 90 pounds of fat and 10 pounds of muscle, their bodies are radically different . . . even though their scale weights are the same!

The following chart, developed at the University of Wisconsin Medical School, represents an ideal weight that corresponds to a healthy body-fat percentage. Go ahead and calculate your ideal weight.

IDEAL WEIGHT

MEN	HEIGHT	WOMEN
	4'11"	95
	5'0"	100
	5'1"	105
118	5'2"	110
124	5'3"	115
130	5'4"	120
136	5'5"	125
142	5'6"	130
148	5'7"	135
154	5'8"	140
160	5'9"	145
166	5'10"	150
172	5'11"	155
178	6'0"	160
184	6'1"	
190	6'2"	
196	6'3"	
202	6'4"	

Your ideal weight: _____

Don't be discouraged if your scale weight exceeds your ideal weight. That will change. Knowing your ideal weight provides a scientific basis for creating your personal fat budget.

STEP 2: DETERMINE YOUR DAILY CALORIES

Once your ideal weight is estimated, you need to know how many calories you can consume each day to sustain that weight. This depends on your level of physical activity. The more active you are, the more calories you need daily. According to the American College of Sports Medicine and the American Dietetic Association, the following levels of activity provide a guideline for estimating your daily caloric needs.

CALORIES NEEDED PER POUND PER DAY

LEVEL OF ACTIVITY	
Extremely inactive, or sedentary	11
Moderately active, or light activity (*Example:* aerobic exercise 2–3 times a week)	13
Active, or moderate exercise and/or work (*Example:* aerobic exercise 4–5 times a week)	15
Extremely active, or heavy exercise and/or work (*Example:* aerobic exercise 6–7 times a week)	18

Combining ideal weight with the appropriate calorie figure in the preceding chart (ideal weight × calories needed per pound per day) allows you to estimate the number of calories needed daily to maintain that weight. For example, if your ideal weight is 125 pounds and you are moderately active, you need about 1,625 calories daily to sustain that weight. The tables below and on the following page provide total calories needed per day by women and men.

CALORIES NEEDED DAILY TO SUSTAIN WEIGHT

WOMEN	IDEAL WEIGHT	INACTIVE	MODERATE	ACTIVE	VERY ACTIVE
4'11"	95	1,045	1,235	1,425	1,710
5'0"	100	1,100	1,300	1,500	1,800
5'1"	105	1,155	1,365	1,575	1,890
5'2"	110	1,210	1,430	1,650	1,980
5'3"	115	1,265	1,495	1,725	2,070
5'4"	120	1,320	1,560	1,800	2,160
5'5"	125	1,375	1,625	1,875	2,250
5'6"	130	1,430	1,690	1,950	2,340
5'7"	135	1,485	1,755	2,025	2,430
5'8"	140	1,540	1,820	2,100	2,520
5'9"	145	1,595	1,885	2,175	2,610
5'10"	150	1,650	1,950	2,250	2,700
5'11"	155	1,705	2,015	2,325	2,790
6'0"	160	1,760	2,080	2,400	2,880

Total calories you need every day: _____

MEN	IDEAL WEIGHT	INACTIVE	MODERATE	ACTIVE	VERY ACTIVE
5'2"	118	1,298	1,534	1,770	2,124
5'3"	124	1,364	1,612	1,860	2,232
5'4"	130	1,430	1,690	1,950	2,340
5'5"	136	1,496	1,768	2,040	2,448
5'6"	142	1,562	1,846	2,130	2,556
5'7"	148	1,628	1,924	2,220	2,664
5'8"	154	1,694	2,002	2,310	2,772
5'9"	160	1,760	2,080	2,400	2,880
5'10"	166	1,826	2,158	2,490	2,988
5'11"	172	1,892	2,236	2,580	3,096
6'0"	178	1,958	2,314	2,670	3,204
6'1"	184	2,024	2,392	2,760	3,312
6'2"	190	2,090	2,470	2,850	3,420
6'3"	196	2,156	2,548	2,940	3,528
6'4"	202	2,222	2,626	3,030	3,636

Total calories you need every day: _____

STEP 3: FIGURE YOUR FAT BUDGET

The accepted guideline is a diet in which fat makes up no more than 30% of total calories. But many experts have observed that this guideline is too high, particularly for those whose aims include weight loss and/or cholesterol reduction.

For most people, a 20% goal is the most effective.

The following table illustrates fat budgets at levels of 15%, 20%, 25% and 30%. Select the goal that best suits your particular needs. (Note that the table begins at 1,200 calories, since it is not recommended that women eat less than 1,200 calories or that men eat fewer than 1,500 calories to meet their daily nutritional needs.)

GRAMS OF FAT ALLOWED

DAILY CALORIE INTAKE	PERCENTAGE OF CALORIES FROM FAT			
	15%	20%	25%	30%
1,200	20	27	33	40
1,300	22	29	36	43
1,400	23	31	39	47
1,500	25	33	42	50
1,600	26	36	44	53
1,700	28	38	47	57
1,800	30	40	50	60
1,900	31	42	53	63
2,000	33	44	56	67
2,100	35	47	58	70
2,200	36	49	61	73
2,300	38	51	64	77
2,400	40	53	67	80
2,500	41	56	69	83
2,600	43	58	72	87
2,700	45	60	75	90
2,800	46	62	77	93
2,900	48	64	80	96
3,000	50	67	83	100

Your personal fat budget: _____ grams

Whichever level you choose, keep in mind that gradual change offers the most potential for success. Give yourself time to adapt to a new way of eating. Small steps over time add up to healthier dietary habits.

USE THE RESTAURANT GUIDE

Once your fat budget is established, the next thing to do is use the restaurant guide to make smarter food choices. It will help to keep you on a lean, healthy diet, yet allow for favorite foods.

This is the way it works. Let's say your budget is 40 grams of fat per day. (Remember, the budget is a *maximum* amount. It's better to eat less.) You start the day with that many grams of fat in your "account." (Think in terms of a checkbook.) As you make your food choices throughout the day, you "spend" your budget. (Think of it as writing a check.)

As long as you stay within your budget, you'll meet the prescription for a low-fat day. By using this book, you'll quickly learn which restaurant foods will—and will not—fit your budget. Having a sandwich on the run? Subway's 6" Club (5 grams of fat) or Boston Market's Ham Sandwich (9 grams of fat) would certainly fit a 40-gram budget. But Arby's Philly Beef 'N Swiss (47 grams) or a generic deli Reuben sandwich (50 grams) would break the bank.

Want to eat pasta for dinner? In most Italian restaurants, an order of pasta with marina sauce is just 5 grams of fat; with red clam sauce, 9 grams; and with meat sauce, 11 grams. Any would fit easily a 40-gram budget. But an order of pasta in a cream sauce, such as Fettucine Alfredo at about 60 grams of fat, would be more than your budget for the entire day.

Luckily, today there is a wider range of lower-fat foods available in sit-down and fast-food restaurants. You simply have to know which items are rich in fat and which are not, and how they fit your budget. With the fat content listed for over 3,500 items, this book in effect provides you with labels for restaurant foods. Now you can learn the fat content of various restaurant foods *before* you order, which will put you in a better position to balance good food with good health.

This guide is divided into two main sections. The first deals with foods offered at **sit-down restaurants**. These foods generally differ from homemade versions in terms of ingredients, preparation and cooking methods. They also can greatly differ in portion size. According to the USDA, for example, the average serving of London broil (flank steak) at home is about 4 ounces, or some 15 grams of fat. But in a restaurant the average serving is about 8 ounces, or over 30 grams of fat. And that doesn't include any fat added in a sauce. Food items even change from restaurant to restaurant. Sometimes portion size is dictated simply by the size of the plates on which the food is served. Moreover, one restaurant might "dry-grill" an item, while another fries it in butter.

Recognizing these variances, we used data from the American Restaurant Association, *Restaurants and Institutions* magazine, individual restaurants and the American Culinary Institute to create a list of the most popular and frequently ordered restaurant foods, their normal serving size and the average fat contained in a serving. Obviously, the list is neither endless nor 100% exact. A chicken breast fillet served at your favorite local restaurant may not match up perfectly to our average, but it will be close enough to give you a good idea of how that food item impacts your budget.

The second section of this guide deals with **fast-food restaurants**. Nutritional information has been supplied by the individual food chains. Because most fast foods are precisely measured, there is a high degree of consistency in fat content. Order a Double Whopper at a Burger King in Seattle or Atlanta and you'll get the same thing—in this instance, 56 grams of fat. A Taco Bell Beef Burrito has 19 grams of fat whether you buy and eat it in Washington, D.C., or in Los Angeles. So, from a monitoring standpoint, fast foods are very consistent and make fat-budgeting easy. *Be aware that fast-food menus change frequently as items are added and deleted.* This guide may not have every item currently offered at a given fast-food restaurant. However, most fast-food restaurant chains maintain a "core" menu (McDonald's will *always* offer a Big Mac, for instance), and it is on these foods that we focus.

It should also be noted that in most instances the figures for calories and fat have been rounded up or down for ease of calculation. If a food has 88 to 92 calories, its caloric content is expressed in the lists as "90 calories"; if it contains 93 to 97 calories, the content is shown as "95 calories." Fat-grams are rounded off to the nearest whole number. If a food item contains less than .5 grams of fat per serving, its fat content is expressed as "0 grams."

ABBREVIATIONS

avg	= average	pkt	= packet
dia	= diameter	sm	= small
lb	= pound	tbsp	= tablespoon
lg	= large	tsp	= teaspoon
med	= medium	w/	= with
oz	= ounce	w/o	= without
pc	= piece	"	= inch
pkg	= package		

RESTAURANT STRATEGIES

Whether you're feasting leisurely at a four-star restaurant or rushing through your favorite fast-food outlet, there are a number of strategies that are important to controlling fat.

KNOW YOUR PERSONAL FAT BUDGET

Your budget is a guideline for the day. Make a point of knowing how many grams of fat you have to "spend" before you go to the restaurant. Don't look on restaurant eating as being distinct from your at-home efforts to stay within your budget. Instead, see it as an extension of those efforts. Develop a healthy mind-set. Don't think of eating out as a "special occasion" to eat whatever you want until you're stuffed. Understand how restaurant foods fit in with your overall dietary plan. And if you do go overboard and exceed your budget, redouble your efforts the following day—take a longer walk when you exercise, for example, and make sure all your meals are really low in fat. You can't undo the high-fat restaurant meal, but you can bring your dietary life back into balance so that your budget evens out.

KNOW HOW MUCH FAT COMES IN RESTAURANT FOODS

Use this book to learn the fat content of your favorite restaurant items so you can preplan your meal before you arrive at the restaurant. There will be less temptation to deviate, you'll get what you want and you'll stay within your budget. If you're in the mood for a burger, for example, you can go to Jack in the Box and order the Jumbo Jack with Cheese, Super Scoop French Fries and a regular chocolate shake for a total of 1,870 calories and 96 grams of fat. Or, using this book to make better choices, you can order a hamburger, regular fries and an orange juice—for a saving of 1,265 calories and 72 grams of fat! Either way, you'll have a burger. But while the first meal is a fat disaster, the second meal does minimal fat-damage. The food lists are a key to balancing your budget and your desires.

CHOOSE A RESTAURANT CAREFULLY

When someone asks "Where do you want to eat?" have in mind a list of restaurants where you're certain you can get low-fat items. Know which restaurants work for you. If you do not, your options might be severely limited. It's more difficult to make low-fat choices, for instance, at a restaurant that specializes in oversize portions of prime rib.

RECOGNIZE THAT FAVORITE FOODS ARE EATEN OVER AND OVER

Research shows that while we might read an entire menu and listen attentively to the daily specials, most people choose the same favorite restaurant foods over and over again. If you like pasta, for example, use this guide to identify those sauces that will not break your budget, such as linguine in a red clam sauce. Think about what you want to order before you get to the restaurant. This will keep you from being caught off guard and ending up with a high-fat meal.

DON'T SET YOURSELF UP TO OVEREAT

If you skip meals all day long to "save calories" for a restaurant dinner, chances are good that you'll overeat. You'll arrive at the restaurant famished, so your resistance to fatty foods will be low. It's also easy to rationalize extras when you're starving. The smarter way is to eat a low-fat breakfast and lunch to compensate for the increased fat at dinner—but be sure to eat. A good tip is to be a little full before you order. You might want to have a glass of mineral water or fruit juice, a piece of fruit, or some raw vegetables and salsa an hour or so before dinner to take the edge off your hunger. Be sure to drink plenty of water during the day—at least five glasses. This keeps your body hydrated and helps to control hunger. Also, watch out for alcohol. It doesn't contain fat, but it may enhance your hunger.

SIT-DOWN RESTAURANTS

S it-down restaurants offer a variety of foods and preparation methods that can work to your benefit in restricting fat. Most restaurants want to please their customers and will make adjustments to lower the fat content of their meals.

GENERAL TIPS

- Make basic low-fat choices. Seafood, for example, is usually lower in fat than red meat; a tomato-based sauce has less fat than a cream-based sauce. Fried foods have more fat than broiled foods. Watch for fatty add-ons such as creamy sauces and dressings. Practice portion control. And learn to distinguish high- from low-fat items on the menu.

- When ordering your meal, consider preparation methods. Ask questions about how a food is prepared. Is it grilled? Fried? Steamed? Are fats added—oil, butter, cream or sour cream? The way to keep salmon from being served in a butter sauce, or vegetables made with melted cheese, is to tell the server what you want—and what you don't want. You, as the customer, have the final say in what you eat. Have your chicken, fish or meat grilled, broiled, baked, roasted or steamed.

- Ask for substitutions to lower fat levels. Requesting a plain baked potato with spicy salsa instead of French fries, for instance, will save 12 grams of fat. Other good substitutions are steamed vegetables for butter-topped and white or brown rice for rice pilaf.

- Look for key words on the menu. *Avoid the following:* buttery, butter sauce, sautéed, fried, pan-fried, crispy, creamed, cream sauce, aioli, pesto, in its own gravy, au gratin, in cheese sauce, escalloped, au lait, à la mode, au fromage, marinated, basted, prime, béarnaise, beurre blanc, Hollandaise. *Choose instead:* steamed, in broth, in its own juice, poached, garden fresh, roasted, broiled, stir-fried, lean.

- Watch for fatty add-ons. Sandwiches made with mayonnaise at home usually contain 1 teaspoon per slice of bread, according to USDA. But restaurants often slather mayonnaise on their sandwiches. If it's more than a thin spread, the sandwich may contain 1 to 1½ tablespoons. And remember, 1 tablespoon of mayonnaise contains 11 grams of fat! Skip creamy sauces and dressings, or have them served on the side. Most cream-based sauces contain 9 to 13 grams of fat per 2 tablespoons. Keep fat levels down by controlling the amount of sauce or dressing you use.

- Practice portion control. Remember, even if your order is low in fat, restaurant portions are generally twice what you'd eat at home. If you order beef, ask for the "petite," "queen" or "8-ounce" portion rather than the "king" or "16-ounce" cut. A good rule of thumb is that the recommended portion of meat or fish—4 ounces—is about the same size as the palm of a woman's hand or a deck of cards or an audiotape (not a videotape!). Four ounces of chicken is about one-half of a chicken breast.

- Salad dressing ladles at salad bars generally hold from 2 to 6 tablespoons of salad dressing. At the high end, that's enough dressing to equal the fat and calories of a burger and fries. And finally, most pasta dishes are calculated on a 9-ounce portion size: a 5-ounce portion of cooked pasta (visualize about 1 cup) and a 4-ounce portion of sauce (visualize about ½ cup). When is the last time a dish of pasta this size was served to you in a restaurant? Most restaurants actually serve 1½ to 2 times that amount. When eaten in too great a quantity, even low-fat foods can add up to excessive fat.

- The "normal" serving size in a restaurant is generally twice what you should be eating. Consider sharing—one person can order an entrée while the other takes the salad bar. If you order a rich dessert, split it. One piece of chocolate cake shared among four people will give everyone a taste without destroying anyone's fat budget. And finally, don't be compelled to eat everything just because you paid for it. Enjoy what you eat, but resist the urge to join the "Clean Plate Club."

SMARTER ORDERING

APPETIZERS

Stay away from appetizers that are fried or deep-fried, drenched in oil, butter or cheese, or served with creamy dips. Nachos with guacamole, deep-fried mozzarella sticks, meat and cheese antipasto, egg rolls, tempura vegetables, buffalo wings and fried calamari are good examples. Start off your meal with a fried whole onion with dipping sauce, for instance, and you take in almost 55 grams of fat—more than you'd get from two Pizza Hut Personal Pan Pepperoni Pizzas. Or eat an order of cheese fries (a pound of French fries covered with cheese and bacon, and served with ranch dressing) and you'll take in 3,000 calories and over 150 grams of fat! Instead, opt for oysters (raw, baked or steamed); steamed mussels; clam, crab, oyster and lobster cocktails; seviche; steamed pot stickers; sushi and sashimi; and steamed or raw vegetables.

SOUPS

Skip cream-based soups, such as clam chowder, and meat soups. Instead, order gazpacho, minestrone, vegetable soup, beef or chicken consommé with pasta or pastina, cioppino and bouillabaisse, and black bean soup.

MEAT, POULTRY AND SEAFOOD

Avoid fatty meat, deep-fried chicken and fish, and foods with fatty sauces and gravies. Ask for meat to be lean, well-trimmed and cooked in a low-fat manner. Order a small piece of sirloin, round steak or London broil, for example, and ask that no oil or butter be used in preparation. Order meat done "medium" or "well-done" to further reduce fat.

Avoid chicken that is fried, batter-dipped and fried, or served smothered in gravy. Order it baked, broiled or barbecued without the skin and with sauces served on the side. If your chicken is served with the skin on, remove the skin before eating. Be aware that roasted turkey dinners with gravy and stuffing can break your fat budget.

Watch out for fish and chips, and any seafood that is fried, deep-fried, breaded and fried, batter-dipped and fried, in a creamy sauce, served with cheese sauce, en casserole, Newburg, Thermidor, baked, stuffed, or stuffed and rolled. Better choices are seafood that is broiled, blackened (Cajun-style), in marinara sauce, in light wine sauce, grilled, barbecued, stir-fried or steamed.

Skip fatty condiments such as butter, drawn butter, mayonnaise, tartar sauce and dill sauce. Better choices are low-sodium soy sauce, lemon juice, wine or vermouth, flavored vinegars and tomato salsa.

SALADS

At the salad bar, skip high-fat extras such as bacon bits, cold cuts, olives, and creamy pasta salad and potato salad. A typical 2-cup salad with all the high-fat extras can have as much fat as a cheeseburger.

A simple green salad is virtually fat-free and runs about 10 calories per ounce. But pour on a couple of table-spoons of dressing and fat/calories soar. Ask for diet and fat-free salad dress-ings. If only a full-fat dressing is avail-able, order it "on the side" and dip your fork in the dressing—you'll get all the flavor but very little of the fat. Don't overlook salsa as an alternative nonfat dressing.

Avoid salads with strips of meat and cheese. Chef's salad—made with cheese, eggs, ham, roast beef and turkey roll, bound together in a creamy dressing— can have 800 calories and 65 grams of fat.

VEGETABLES

Avoid vegetables prepared or topped with butter, cream, cheese, cheese sauce or oil. Instead, ask for sodium-reduced soy sauce, flavored vinegars, lemon juice and hot sauce to flavor vegetables without fat. Order fresh vegetables such as asparagus, broccoli and mushrooms, either raw or slightly steamed. Potatoes, rice and noodles are low in fat when prepared or served without butter, sour cream and other fatty condiments.

DESSERTS

Limit commercial pastries, pies, cakes, cookies and candies. Fresh fruit, nonfat yogurt, gelatine, sherbet, sorbet, ices and unfrosted angel food cake are smarter choices. If you choose to eat a rich dessert, share it with others.

BREAKFASTS

Avoid fatty meats, whole eggs, fried foods and sugared cereals. Watch out for the breakfast buffet; not only does it contain an array of fatty foods (sausages, eggs, hash browns), but it also offers as much as you can eat—a dangerous combination. Instead, center your meal on low-fat cereals, muffins or toast, juice and fresh fruit. If you do order eggs, have them poached, boiled or shirred, but not fried. If you can't do without breakfast meat, Canadian bacon is preferable to sausage, bacon and ham.

ETHNIC FOODS

ITALIAN

In Italian restaurants, choose vegetable antipasto (roasted peppers and zucchini, grilled mushrooms); minestrone soup, ribollito (thick vegetable stew) and cioppino (seafood stew); pasta with meatless tomato-based sauces such as marinara, light red, pomodoro, vegetable and red seafood sauce; pasta e fagioli (shells and beans); grilled game, veal and fish; veal piccata (sautéed in lemon juice); scampi sautéed in wine; baked or broiled chicken; chicken cacciatore; fish dishes topped with meatless tomato sauce and little or no cheese; Italian ice or fruit for dessert.

It's better to go easy or avoid meat (sausage, pepperoni, mortadella) and cheese antipasto; garlic bread (made with butter or oil); fried calamari; bruschetta (bread drenched in olive oil); pasta in butter, cheese, oil, cream or bacon fat (pancetta), such as Alfredo or carbonara sauces, as well as those made with pesto or sausage; cheese- and meat-stuffed pasta dishes (tortellini, ravioli, cannelloni, manicotti, lasagna); frito misto (a fried mix of seafood, meat and vegetables); risotto (heavy with butter and cheese); cheesy eggplant or veal parmigiana; veal piccata (sautéed in butter) and veal marsala; rich desserts such as tiramisu or cannoli. If you order pizza, hold the meat, go easy on the cheese and double the vegetables.

MEXICAN/SOUTHWESTERN

The best choices are Mexican/Southwestern foods that stick to the basics: mesquite-grilled chicken, seafood and lean cuts of beef or pork; chili con carne; enchiladas, burritos and soft-shell tacos (unfried) with chicken, seafood and vegetable fillings (hold the sour cream and cheese); and black bean soup and gazpacho.

Watch out for tortilla chips and nachos; deep-fried and fried dishes such as chimichangas, flautas and taquitos; crispy taco or salad shells; quesadillas; cheese dishes such as chili con queso; refried beans made with lard; fatty "extras" such as cheese, sour cream and guacamole; dishes with poblano aioli (chili mayonnaise) or cilantro pesto. Be aware that fajitas and taco salads can contain a surprising amount of fat, and that combination dinners are usually heavy in fat and calories.

FRENCH/CONTINENTAL

Choose the foods of southern France, which use seafood, vegetables, wine and olive oil. Smart choices are poached, roasted or broiled fish and chicken (such as coq au vin); lean meats; foods steamed in parchment, or steamed or sautéed in wine; dishes labeled coulis, vegetable puree or reduction; salade Niçoise; consommé; stews such as bouillabaisse or ratatouille.

Go easy on or avoid the foods of northern France, which center on meat, sausage, goose, lard, goose fat, butter, cream and fatty sauces; cassoulet and gratins (made with cheese or egg); dishes heavy with eggs, such as quenelles, soufflés and quiche; goose or duck pâté; organ meats; rich sauces such as béarnaise, buerre blanc, béchamel and Hollandaise; items in a pastry shell; croissants; and pastry.

CHINESE

Chinese food offers a variety of low-fat options. Smarter choices include hot-and-sour wonton soup; steamed dumplings (Chinese raviolis); and roast pork strips. Choose stir-fried or steamed dishes with vegetables, chicken, seafood or tofu; steamed or braised whole fish or scallops; steamed rice. Ask for meals with no added salt or MSG, and with as little oil as possible. One-cup servings with less than 10 grams of fat include hot-and-sour soup, stir-fried vegetables, Szechuan shrimp, lo mein, chicken chow mein and Hunan tofu.

Foods to avoid or go easy on include dishes made with duck, beef and pork (duck dishes are among the highest, so avoid Peking duck and crispy duck); items that have been fried or deep-fried such as egg rolls, dumplings, fried shrimp, fried wontons and fried rice; sweet-and-sour dishes; anything "crispy" or "batter-coated"; and dishes heavy on nuts. Some of the fattest choices include Kung Pao chicken, moo shu pork, sweet-and-sour pork, crispy beef and fried rice.

JAPANESE

Japanese steak houses offer an American version of Japanese food—one that is not low in fat. Authentic Japanese cooking, however, is centered on low-fat rice and vegetables and uses little or no fat in cooking. Dishes to choose include miso soup; sunomono (cucumber salad); yakitori (broiled chicken); Japanese vegetables; chicken and fish teriyaki; hibachi chicken and lean beef, sushi and sashimi; yosenabe (seafood and vegetable stew); shabu-shabu (vegetables and meats boiled in broth); and rice and noodles.

Go easy on or avoid deep-fried foods (tempura, agemono and katsu); sukiyaki; and egg dishes such as oyako-donburi.

THAI

Thai food is generally light in calories and fat. Rice, noodles and vegetables dominate the menu, so it's easy to keep servings of meat and seafood moderate. Choose entrées that are stir-fried, steamed, boiled or barbecued. In addition to vegetables, entrées include shrimp, scallops, squid, clams, chicken, beef and pork.

Avoid duck entrées, they're too fatty. Also, be certain that the restaurant stir-fries in oil, not lard. Watch out for appetizers such as fried or stuffed chicken wings, Thai rolls, tod mum and golden bags, which are fried or deep-fried. Be aware that many dishes contain peanuts, cashews or peanut sauces, which can raise fat content. Avoid dishes made with coconut milk (which has about 48 grams of fat per cup), such as curry or chicken coconut soup. If you do order curry, a Thai specialty, consider sharing it with a friend.

INDIAN

Smarter choices include lentil soups like mulligatawny or dal rasam; yogurt-based curries; chicken or fish prepared tandoori, tikka, vindaloo or masala style.

Go easy on or avoid fried appetizers like samosas and pakoras, and fried breads such as poori and paratha. Watch out for any dishes called malai, kandhari and korma, which are made with cream or coconut.

CAJUN

Choose red beans and rice (without sausage); mustard greens, okra and kale (hold the bacon); chicken or seafood jambalaya or gumbo; shrimp Creole and other tomato-based dishes; blackened fish; and boiled seafood dinners.

Go easy on or avoid hush puppies (fried corn bread); dirty rice (fried rice with sausage or other fatty meats); sausage dishes including boudin or andouille; cream-based soups or bisque; étouffée; and batter-fried seafoods.

APPETIZERS & SNACKS

	AMOUNT	CALORIES	FAT-GRAMS	% FAT
Antipasto platter (salami, prosciutto, cheese, olives, anchovies, egg, tomato, lettuce, onion, celery)	I serving	230	15	59
Artichoke, fresh	I med	55	0	0
Asparagus w/ prosciutto	3 spears	55	2	33
Avocado	½	155	14	81
BBQ pork w/ seeds & hot mustard	2 oz	215	14	59
BBQ ribs	3 oz	390	27	63
Beef Chiang Mai	I serving	125	8	58
Beef, dried	I oz	50	I	18
Belgian pâté	2 oz	150	184	83
Black bean soup w/o sour cream	I cup	115	2	15
Bruschetta (broiled Italian or French bread, olive oil)	I slice	240	20	75
Calamari, fried	5 oz	215	11	48
Caponata	6 oz	185	14	68

	AMOUNT	CALORIES	FAT-GRAMS	% FAT
Caviar	1 tbsp	40	2	43
w/ hard-cooked eggs, chopped onions & chives	1 tbsp	140	5	32
Celery				
stuffed w/ blue cheese	2 stalks	105	9	76
stuffed w/ olives & cream cheese	2 stalks	85	7	74
Cheese:				
Baked chèvre w/ French roll	1 serving	275	11	36
Buffalo mozzarella w/ tomatoes, basil, black olives & olive oil	3 oz	345	37	96
Cheese & crab tarts	2	400	28	63
Cheese cubes	1	105	9	77
Cheese bagel bites	1	30	2	60
Cheese board (2 oz cheese, 2 oz crackers)	1 serving	510	34	59
Cheese fondue	½ cup	305	18	46
Cheese fries	1 cup	595	38	57
w/ ranch dressing	2 tbsp	750	54	66
Cheese nuggets (½-oz balls)	2	165	9	49
Cheese puffs/twists	1 cup	235	15	57
Cheese sticks	1 stick	160	11	62
Cherry tomato stuffed w/ cream cheese	1	35	3	75

	AMOUNT	CALORIES	FAT-GRAMS	% FAT
Crab & cheese tarts	2	400	28	63
Fried cheese				
(2½ × ½ × ½)	I stick	75	5	59
Fried cheese kabob	I	65	4	55
Fried mozzarella w/				
marinara sauce	3 oz	340	22	58
Marinated mozzarella	I oz	150	14	85
Pesto cheese torta				
(pesto, mascarpone,				
ricotta)	2.5 oz	155	13	75
Ricotta cheese spread	I tbsp	45	2	40
Swiss cheese tartlets	2	435	33	68
Chex mix	I oz	180	7	35
Chicken:				
Chicken liver pâté	¼ cup	295	26	79
on 1 slice toast	I serving	160	8	36
Chicken livers				
wrapped in bacon				
(rumaki)	2	105	5	44
Chicken chow mein	I cup	255	10	35
Chopped chicken liver				
& eggs	¼ cup	210	17	72
Chicken nuggets,				
w/o sauce	4	240	14	52
Chicken wings				
BBQ	I	130	6	41
Batter-dipped, fried	I	160	11	62
Cajun	I	130	7	49
Ginger	I	170	13	69
Teriyaki	I	155	6	35

	AMOUNT	CALORIES	FAT-GRAMS	% FAT
Chili:				
Chili con queso	½ cup	400	32	73
w/ 1 oz chips	1 serving	540	38	63
Chili w/ beans	1 cup	300	15	45
Chili w/o beans	1 cup	300	19	57
Chinese crab claws	2	150	8	49
Chips:				
Chips & salsa				
(1 cup chips,				
¼ cup salsa)	1 serving	215	11	51
Corn chips	1 oz	150	10	60
Nacho chips	1 oz	150	8	48
Potato chips	1 oz	150	10	60
Taco chips	1 oz	140	7	47
Tortilla chips	1 oz	140	6	38
w/ ¼ cup salsa	1 serving	160	7	39
Nachos, cheese				
(1 oz chips, 2 oz sauce)	1 serving	310	13	38
Nachos, deluxe				
(1 oz chips, 2 oz sauce,				
ground beef, refried				
beans, cheese)	1 serving	430	19	40
Nachos Grande				
(2 oz chips, ground				
beef, tomatoes,				
olives, cheese,				
lettuce, sour cream)	1 serving	635	39	55
Cheese puffs/twists	1 cup	235	15	57
Chop suey w/ beef				
& pork	1 cup	300	17	51

	AMOUNT	CALORIES	FAT-GRAMS	% FAT
Clams				
Clam fritter	1.5 oz	125	6	44
Clams on half-shell	6	150	1	6
Deviled clams	1 ramekin	360	14	35
Fried clams	6 oz	380	20	47
Steamed clams				
(in shells)	1 lb	265	8	28
w/ olive oil & lemon		335	21	56
Cocktail meatballs	3	150	9	54
Codfish balls	1	50	3	55
Corn & cheese chowder	¾ cup	215	12	50
Corn nuts	1 cup	375	12	29
Crab:				
Chinese crab claws	2	150	8	49
Crab cake	1	160	10	56
Crab & cheese tarts	2	400	28	63
Crab claws	6 oz	145	1	6
Crab Imperial	1 ramekin	140	7	44
Crabmeat cocktail	1 serving	130	2	14
Crab pillows	3	120	6	46
Crab, soft-shell, fried	1	335	18	48
Crab, stuffed	½ cup	85	4	42
Crackers:				
Cheese crackers	14	70	4	51
Chicken in a Biskit	7	70	4	51
Cracked wheat				
crackers	4	110	4	33
Crispbread crackers	3	60	2	30
Hearty wheat				
crackers	4	100	4	36

	AMOUNT	CALORIES	FAT-GRAMS	% FAT
Lahvosh	1	30	1	30
Melba toast cracker	1	20	0	0
Milk crackers	1	55	2	33
Oyster crackers	16	60	2	30
Ritz crackers	4	70	4	51
Rye crisps	4	90	0	0
Saltines	2	25	1	36
Triscuits	7	145	5	31
Toasted sesame cracker	1	30	0	0
Water biscuit	3	90	3	30
Wheatsworth crackers	5	70	3	38
Wheat thins	7	80	4	45
Dips:				
Avocado	¼ cup	100	8	72
Bacon & horseradish	¼ cup	100	10	90
Blue cheese	¼ cup	125	9	65
Clam dip	¼ cup	140	10	63
Creamy cucumber	¼ cup	100	8	72
French onion	¼ cup	120	8	60
Garlic	¼ cup	120	8	60
Guacamole	¼ cup	80	8	88
Jalapeño	¼ cup	120	10	75
Nacho cheese	¼ cup	100	4	36
Picante sauce	¼ cup	40	0	0
Egg rolls:				
Crab-filled	1	155	10	58
Ham-filled	1	135	8	54
Meatless	1	100	6	52
Pork-filled	1	170	8	42

	AMOUNT	CALORIES	FAT-GRAMS	% FAT
Pork & shrimp-filled	1	160	9	51
Shrimp-filled	1	190	6	29
Vegetable-filled	1	120	6	45
Eggs:				
Deviled	1 egg	140	12	77
Pickled	1 egg	85	6	64
Empanadas	2	195	14	64
Escargot w/ butter				
sauce	3 oz	450	25	50
Falafel	1 patty	60	3	45
Finger sandwiches:				
Cheese	1 sq	45	2	40
Cucumber	1 sq	30	1	30
Cucumber & shrimp	1 sq	45	2	40
Ham	1 sq	45	2	40
Watercress	1 sq	45	2	40
Frog's leg, fried	1	70	5	64
Fruit:				
Citrus cocktail	½ cup	55	0	0
w/ avocado		70	2	26
Fruit cocktail	½ cup	65	0	0
Fruit platter				
w/ 2 oz cheese	1 serving	310	18	52
Mandarin orange/				
banana cocktail	½ cup	45	0	0
Melon & prosciutto	1 wedge	35	1	26
Melon cocktail	½ cup	30	0	0
in syrup		85	0	0
Peach & green grape				
cocktail	½ cup	40	0	0

	AMOUNT	CALORIES	FAT-GRAMS	% FAT
Gazpacho	1 cup	45	0	0
Gyoza	4	255	9	32
Ham:				
Ham & cheese spread	1 tbsp	40	3	68
Ham croquettes	1	220	14	57
Ham salad spread	1 tbsp	30	2	60
Ham patty, grilled	1	205	18	79
Ham phyllo roll	1	75	3	36
Herring:				
Kippered	1 fillet	90	5	50
Pickled	1.75 oz	130	6	42
Hot & sour soup	1 cup	75	2	24
Hummus	1 cup	450	22	44
Jambalaya	1 cup	250	7	25
Kielbasa in fondue	6 oz	410	33	72
Lobster				
Cocktail	1 serving	130	2	14
Newburg	6.5 oz	455	35	69
Miso	½ cup	285	8	25
Mushrooms:				
Bread-stuffed	1	35	2	51
Cheese-stuffed	1	45	3	63
Marinated	2	15	1	60
Wrapped in bacon	2	50	4	69
Mushroom spread				
w/ 2 crackers	1 serving	85	2	21
Mussels, steamed				
(in olive oil, garlic,				
tomatoes)	1 doz	330	12	33
Nachos. *See* Chips.				

	AMOUNT	CALORIES	FAT-GRAMS	% FAT
Nuts:				
Almonds				
Dry roasted	1 oz	170	15	80
Honey roasted	1 oz	170	13	69
Cashews	1 oz	170	13	69
Macadamia nuts	1 oz	200	21	95
Mixed nuts	1 oz	170	13	69
Peanuts				
Dry roasted	1 oz	160	14	79
Honey roasted	1 oz	160	13	73
Oil roasted	1 oz	170	15	79
Pistachios	1 oz	170	15	79
Oxtail soup	5 oz	65	3	42
Olives:				
Green				
Medium	10	45	5	100
Large	10	65	7	100
Giant	10	75	8	100
Ripe (extra-large)	10	60	6	100
Stuffed, rolled w/ bacon	2	50	4	75
Onions:				
Fried whole	1 cup	565	39	62
w/ dipping sauce	2 tbsp	710	54	68
Rings	8	275	16	52
Oysters:				
Angels on horseback (oysters wrapped in bacon)	1	60	4	61
Oysters battered & fried	6	370	18	44
Oysters on half-shell	6	120	2	15

	AMOUNT	CALORIES	FAT-GRAMS	% FAT
Oysters Rockefeller	6	355	26	66
Oyster shooter	l med	40	1	22
Oyster stew	l cup	280	18	58
Paella	8 oz	350	11	28
Pâté:				
Belgian pâté	2 oz	150	14	83
Chicken liver pâté	¼ cup	295	26	79
Goose liver pâté	l oz	130	12	82
Pepperoni	l oz	110	10	82
Pierogi	¾ cup	310	19	55
Piroshki:				
Ham & egg	2	320	23	64
Russian	2	340	24	64
Pizza bites	2 pcs	65	4	55
Pizza bread				
(1 slice bread,				
1 oz cheese)	l serving	200	10	45
Popcorn:				
Air-popped	l cup	30	0	0
Coated w/ sugar syrup	l cup	135	1	7
Oil-popped	l cup	55	3	49
w/ ½ tsp butter		70	5	62
Pork rinds	l oz	115	7	55
Potatoes:				
Cheese fries	l cup	595	38	57
w/ ranch dressing	2 tbsp	750	54	66
French fries	l reg serving	235	12	46
	l lg serving	355	19	48
Fried potato skins	l reg serving	220	12	50
Potato chips	l oz	150	10	60

	AMOUNT	CALORIES	FAT GRAMS	% FAT
Potato puffs	1	15	1	60
Potato sticks	1 oz	190	12	57
Spiral fries	1 reg serving	285	14	44
Pot stickers	4	255	9	32
Pretzels	1 oz	110	1	8
Rice cake	1	35	0	0
Rumaki	2	105	5	44
Salami, hard	1 oz	100	9	90
Salmon:				
Salmon cake	1	240	15	56
Smoked salmon w/ 2 oz cream cheese, capers, onions	3 oz	100	4	36
Salsa	2 tbsp	10	0	0
Sardines:				
Sardines in oil	2	50	3	54
Sardines in tomato sauce	1	70	5	64
Sauerkraut balls	2	120	5	37
Sausage:				
Bratwurst	1 oz	90	8	80
Italian sausage	1 oz	90	7	70
Kielbasa sausage	1 oz	90	8	80
Sausage roll	1	310	24	70
Vienna sausage	2 oz	125	10	72
Scallops, fried	2 lg	70	3	39
Seafood gumbo	5 oz	50	1	18
Seafood nuggets	2 oz	130	8	55
Shrimp:				
BBQ jumbo shrimp	4 lg	70	1	13
Breaded & fried shrimp	4 lg	75	4	48

	AMOUNT	CALORIES	FAT GRAMS	% FAT
Curried shrimp	¾ cup	230	12	47
Jumbo prawn cocktail	6 prawns	155	2	12
Peel & eat shrimp	3 oz	90	1	10
Shrimp cocktail	4 shrimp	105	1	9
Shrimp Creole	1 cup	300	9	27
Shrimp stew	1 cup	210	14	60
Shrimp wrapped in bacon	1 shrimp	30	2	60
Soup:				
Black bean soup w/o sour cream	1 cup	115	2	15
Corn & cheese chowder	¾ cup	215	12	50
Gazpacho	1 cup	45	0	0
Hot & sour soup	1 cup	75	2	24
Jambalaya	1 cup	250	7	25
Miso	½ cup	285	8	25
Oxtail soup	5 oz	65	3	42
Oyster stew	1 cup	280	18	58
Seafood gumbo	5 oz	50	1	18
Shrimp stew	1 cup	210	14	60
Spring rolls, fried	1	130	8	55
Squash blossoms stuffed w/ prosciutto, mozzarella & ricotta	4	170	12	64
Steak tartare	4 oz	545	39	64
Sweet & sour pork	¾ cup	190	8	38
Sushi:				
California roll	1	30	1	30
Sashimi	6 oz	200	7	32
Tuna roll	1	30	1	30

	AMOUNT	CALORIES	FAT GRAMS	% FAT
Vegetable roll	1	30	1	30
Yellowtail roll	1	25	1	36
Szechuan pork & seeds				
w/ hot mustard	2 oz	215	14	59
Tuna:				
Broiled tuna Hawaiian				
on 1 slice bread	1 serving	105	6	52
Deviled tuna				
cheeseburger				
(petite bun)	1 serving	235	11	42
Patty	3 oz	230	8	31
Turkey:				
Aiguillettes	2 oz	210	13	56
Sticks, breaded & fried	5 oz	400	24	54
Vegetable antipasto				
platter, marinated	1 serving	255	20	80
Vegetables:				
Batter-fried	¾ cup	150	7	42
Raw w/ olive oil	1 serving	225	20	80
Welsh rarebit	1 cup	415	32	69
Wontons, filled	4	255	9	32
w/ pork, fried	1	80	4	45
Wonton skins, fried	½ cup	110	8	65
Zucchini carpaccio	1 serving	280	27	87

BEVERAGES

	AMOUNT	CALORIES	FAT-GRAMS	% FAT
ALCOHOLIC BEVERAGES				
Beer, Ale & Malt Liquor				
Ale, brown	10 fl oz	80	0	0
Ale, pale	10 fl oz	90	0	0
Beer	12 fl oz	145	0	0
Beer, light	12 fl oz	100	0	0
Lager	10 fl oz	80	0	0
Malt Liquor	12 fl oz	150	0	0
Stout	10 fl oz	100	0	0
Amstel Light	12 fl oz	95	0	0
Anheuser-Busch	12 fl oz	155	0	0
Anheuser-Busch				
Natural Light	12 fl oz	110	0	0
Beck's	12 fl oz	145	0	0
Beck's Dark	12 fl oz	155	0	0
Black Horse	12 fl oz	160	0	0
Black Label	12 fl oz	135	0	0
Blatz Ale	12 fl oz	155	0	0
Blatz Beer	12 fl oz	140	0	0
Budweiser	12 fl oz	145	0	0
Bud Light	12 fl oz	110	0	0
Busch	12 fl oz	145	0	0

	AMOUNT	CALORIES	FAT-GRAMS	% FAT
Busch Light	12 fl oz	100	0	0
Carlsberg	12 fl oz	150	0	0
Carlsberg Light	12 fl oz	110	0	0
Champale Malt Liquor	12 fl oz	170	0	0
Colt 45 Malt Liquor	12 fl oz	155	0	0
Coors	12 fl oz	140	0	0
Coors Dry	12 fl oz	120	0	0
Coors Extra Gold	12 fl oz	150	0	0
Coors Light	12 fl oz	105	0	0
Corona Light	12 fl oz	105	0	0
Hamm's	12 fl oz	140	0	0
Hamm's Light	12 fl oz	95	0	0
Heidelberg Light	12 fl oz	115	0	0
Heileman Old Style	12 fl oz	145	0	0
Heileman Light	12 fl oz	100	0	0
Heileman Special Export	12 fl oz	155	0	0
Heileman Special Export Light	12 fl oz	115	0	0
Heineken	12 fl oz	150	0	0
Killian's	12 fl oz	160	0	0
Killian's 3.2%	12 fl oz	130	0	0
Knickerbocker	12 fl oz	140	0	0
LA	12 fl oz	115	0	0
Lite Genuine Draft	12 fl oz	100	0	0
Lite "Lite"	12 fl oz	95	0	0
Löwenbrau Dark Special	12 fl oz	160	0	0
Löwenbrau Special	12 fl oz	160	0	0
Meister Brau	12 fl oz	140	0	0

	AMOUNT	CALORIES	FAT-GRAMS	% FAT
Meister Brau Light	12 fl oz	100	0	0
Michelob	12 fl oz	160	0	0
Michelob Classic Dark	12 fl oz	165	0	0
Michelob Dry	12 fl oz	135	0	0
Michelob Light	12 fl oz	135	0	0
Mickey's Malt Liquor	12 fl oz	155	0	0
Miller Genuine Draft	12 fl oz	150	0	0
Miller High Life	12 fl oz	150	0	0
Miller Lite	12 fl oz	95	0	0
Milwaukee's Best	12 fl oz	135	0	0
Milwaukee's Best Light	12 fl oz	100	0	0
Molson Light	12 fl oz	110	0	0
Olde English Malt Liquor	12 fl oz	165	0	0
Old Milwaukee	12 fl oz	145	0	0
Old Milwaukee Light	12 fl oz	120	0	0
Old Style Light	12 fl oz	115	0	0
Olympia	12 fl oz	145	0	0
Olympia Gold Light	12 fl oz	70	0	0
Pabst Blue Ribbon	12 fl oz	145	0	0
Pabst Blue Ribbon Light	12 fl oz	70	0	0
Piels Light	12 fl oz	135	0	0
Rainier	12 fl oz	140	0	0
Rheingold	12 fl oz	150	0	0
Rheingold Light	12 fl oz	95	0	0
Rolling Rock Premium	12 fl oz	145	0	0
Rolling Rock Light	12 fl oz	105	0	0
Schaefer	12 fl oz	140	0	0
Schaefer Light	12 fl oz	110	0	0

	AMOUNT	CALORIES	FAT-GRAMS	% FAT
Schaefer Malt Liquor	12 fl oz	165	0	0
Schlitz	12 fl oz	145	0	0
Schlitz Light	12 fl oz	95	0	0
Schlitz Malt Liquor	12 fl oz	180	0	0
Schmidt's	12 fl oz	150	0	0
Schmidt's Light	12 fl oz	95	0	0
Stroh's	12 fl oz	145	0	0
Stroh's Light	12 fl oz	115	0	0
Tiger Head Ale	12 fl oz	165	0	0
Zima	12 fl oz	150	0	0

Distilled Liquor

(Bourbon, gin, rum, rye whiskey, scotch, tequila, vodka, & whiskey. The higher the proof, the greater the amount of alcohol and calories.)

Proof				
80	1 fl oz	67	0	0
84	1 fl oz	70	0	0
86	1 fl oz	72	0	0
90	1 fl oz	75	0	0
94	1 fl oz	78	0	0
97	1 fl oz	81	0	0
100	1 fl oz	83	0	0
Bloody Mary	5 fl oz	120	0	0
Bourbon & soda	5 fl oz	120	0	0
Brandy Alexander	5 fl oz	275	9	29
Brandy cream	4 fl oz	150	7	42
Campari & soda	5 fl oz	120	0	0

	AMOUNT	CALORIES	FAT-GRAMS	% FAT
Daiquiri:	2.5 fl oz	90	0	0
Banana	4 fl oz	145	0	0
Peach	4 fl oz	110	0	0
Strawberry	4 fl oz	145	0	0
Gin:				
90-proof	1 jigger	110	0	0
94-proof	1 jigger	115	0	0
100-proof	1 jigger	125	0	0
Gin & tonic	7.5 fl oz	170	0	0
Gin ricky	4 fl oz	150	0	0
Glogg	4 fl oz	190	2	9
Golden Cadillac	4 fl oz	230	7	27
Grasshopper	4 fl oz	230	7	27
Highball	7.5 fl oz	165	0	0
Manhattan	2 fl oz	130	0	0
Margarita	7 fl oz	160	0	0
Martini	2.5 fl oz	155	0	0
Mint julep	10 fl oz	210	0	0
Old-fashioned	2.5 fl oz	130	0	0
Piña colada	4.5 fl oz	260	3	10
Rum:				
80-proof	1 jigger	100	0	0
94-proof	1 jigger	115	0	0
100-proof	1 jigger	125	0	0
Scotch	1 jigger	115	0	0
Screwdriver	7 fl oz	175	0	0
Sloe gin fizz	2.5 fl oz	130	0	0
Tequila	1 jigger	115	0	0
Tequila Sunrise	5 fl oz	200	0	0
Tom Collins	5 fl oz	120	0	0

	AMOUNT	CALORIES	FAT-GRAMS	% FAT
Velvet Hammer	4 fl oz	230	7	27
Vodka:				
94-proof	1 jigger	115	0	0
100-proof	1 jigger	125	0	0
Whiskey:				
94-proof	1 jigger	115	0	0
100-proof	1 jigger	125	0	0
Whiskey sour	4 fl oz	170	0	0
Liqueurs				
Anisette	1 fl oz	100	0	0
Apricot brandy	1 fl oz	80	0	0
B&B	1 fl oz	95	0	0
Benedictine	1 fl oz	95	0	0
Campari	1.5 fl oz	120	0	0
Cherry Heering	1.5 fl oz	120	0	0
Coffee liqueur:				
53-proof	1.5 fl oz	175	0	0
63-proof	1.5 fl oz	160	0	0
Coffee w/ Cream	1.5 fl oz	155	0	0
Crème d'Amande	1.5 fl oz	150	0	0
Crème de Banane	1.5 fl oz	145	0	0
Crème de Cacao	1.5 fl oz	150	0	0
Crème de Cassis	1.5 fl oz	120	0	0
Crème de Menthe	1.5 fl oz	190	0	0
Curaçao	1.5 fl oz	110	0	0
Drambuie	1.5 fl oz	165	0	0
Kirsch	1.5 fl oz	125	0	0
Peppermint schnapps	1.5 fl oz	125	0	0

	AMOUNT	CALORIES	FAT-GRAMS	% FAT
Pernod	1.5 fl oz	120	0	0
Sloe Gin	1.5 fl oz	125	0	0
Southern Comfort	1.5 fl oz	180	0	0
Tia Maria	1.5 fl oz	140	0	0
Triple Sec	1.5 fl oz	120	0	0
Wines				
Beaujolais	4 fl oz	95	0	0
Bordeaux, red	4 fl oz	95	0	0
Burgundy:				
Red	4 fl oz	95	0	0
Sparking	4 fl oz	115	0	0
White	4 fl oz	90	0	0
Cabernet Sauvignon	4 fl oz	90	0	0
Chablis:	4 fl oz	85	0	0
Gold, Pink, Emerald	4 fl oz	100	0	0
Champagne:				
Brut, pink	4 fl oz	100	0	0
Extra-dry	4 fl oz	105	0	0
Chardonnay	4 fl oz	90	0	0
Chenin Blanc	4 fl oz	85	0	0
Chianti	4 fl oz	100	0	0
Cold Duck	4 fl oz	110	0	0
Cooking:				
Red, white	½ cup	5	0	0
Sherry	½ cup	40	0	0
Dessert	4 fl oz	180	0	0
Dubonnet	4 fl oz	160	0	0
French Colombard	4 fl oz	90	0	0
Liebfraumilch	4 fl oz	85	0	0

	AMOUNT	CALORIES	FAT-GRAMS	% FAT
Madeira	4 fl oz	160	0	0
Marsala	4 fl oz	80	0	0
Merlot	4 fl oz	95	0	0
Moselle	4 fl oz	100	0	0
Muscatel	3.5 fl oz	160	0	0
Port:				
Ruby, tawny	4 fl oz	185	0	0
White	4 fl oz	170	0	0
Reisling	4 fl oz	90	0	0
Rhine	4 fl oz	95	0	0
Rhone	4 fl oz	95	0	0
Rosé	4 fl oz	95	0	0
Sangría	4 fl oz	115	0	0
Sauterne	4 fl oz	115	0	0
Sauvignon Blanc	4 fl oz	80	0	0
Sherry:				
Cream	4 fl oz	115	0	0
Dry	4 fl oz	110	0	0
Sweet wines	4 fl oz	165	0	0
Sylvaner	4 fl oz	90	0	0
Table wines:				
Red, rosé	3.5 fl oz	75	0	0
White	3.5 fl oz	70	0	0
Tokay	4 fl oz	165	0	0
Vermouth:				
Dry	4 fl oz	135	0	0
Sweet	4 fl oz	170	0	0
Wine cooler, Bartles				
& James	6 fl oz	75	0	0
	12 fl oz	190	0	0

	AMOUNT	CALORIES	FAT-GRAMS	% FAT
Wine spritzer	5 fl oz	60	0	0
Zinfandel:				
Red	4 fl oz	90	0	0
White	4 fl oz	80	0	0

NONALCOHOLIC BEVERAGES

Drink Mixers

	AMOUNT	CALORIES	FAT-GRAMS	% FAT
Bitter lemon	6 fl oz	75	0	0
Club soda	6 fl oz	0	0	0
Collins mixer	6 fl oz	60	0	0
Ginger ale	6 fl oz	70	0	0
Ginger ale, diet	6 fl oz	5	0	0
Grapefruit	6 fl oz	80	0	0
Lemon-lime	6 fl oz	75	0	0
Lemon-lime, diet	6 fl oz	0	0	0
Lemon sour	6 fl oz	75	0	0
Quinine water	6 fl oz	70	0	0
Seltzer, plain & flavored	6 fl oz	0	0	0
Sour mixer	6 fl oz	70	0	0
Tonic water	6 fl oz	65	0	0
Tonic water, diet	6 fl oz	5	0	0
Vodka mixer	6 fl oz	70	0	0
Mineral & bottled water	6 fl oz	0	0	0

Nonalcoholic Beer

	AMOUNT	CALORIES	FAT-GRAMS	% FAT
Cheers	12 fl oz	55	0	0
Guinness Kaliber	12 fl oz	45	0	0
Hamm's	12 fl oz	55	0	0

	AMOUNT	CALORIES	FAT-GRAMS	% FAT
Kingsbury	12 fl oz	60	0	0
Moussy	12 fl oz	50	0	0
Pabst	12 fl oz	55	0	0
Schmidt's	12 fl oz	80	0	0
Sharp's	12 fl oz	75	0	0
Spirit	12 fl oz	80	0	0
Soft Drinks				
Apple	6 fl oz	90	0	0
Apple, diet	6 fl oz	10	0	0
Black cherry	6 fl oz	90	0	0
Black cherry, diet	6 fl oz	5	0	0
Cherry cola	6 fl oz	80	0	0
Cherry cola, diet	6 fl oz	0	0	0
Cherry	6 fl oz	0	0	0
Cola	6 fl oz	80	0	0
Cola, diet	6 fl oz	0	0	0
Cream soda	6 fl oz	95	0	0
Cream soda, diet	6 fl oz	0	0	0
Grape	6 fl oz	90	0	0
Grape, diet	6 fl oz	5	0	0
7-Up	6 fl oz	80	0	0
7-Up, diet	6 fl oz	0	0	0
Orange	6 fl oz	100	0	0
Orange, diet	6 fl oz	5	0	0
Punch:				
Fruit	4 fl oz	65	0	0
Ice cream	4 fl oz	125	4	29
Lime ice ginger ale	4 fl oz	65	0	0
Rhubarb	4 fl oz	120	0	0

	AMOUNT	CALORIES	FAT GRAMS	% FAT
Sherbet	4 fl oz	125	1	7
Slushy	4 fl oz	75	0	0
Slushy, spiked	4 fl oz	100	0	0
Root beer	6 fl oz	85	0	0
Root beer, diet	6 fl oz	0	0	0
Root beer float	12 fl oz	185	7	34
Strawberry	6 fl oz	90	0	0
Strawberry, diet	6 fl oz	0	0	0

Chocolate/Cocoa Drinks
Chocolate/cocoa, hot

	AMOUNT	CALORIES	FAT GRAMS	% FAT
Prepared w/ water	6 fl oz	50	0	0
Diet	6 fl oz	20	0	0
Prepared w/				
Skim milk	6 fl oz	135	2	10
1% milk	6 fl oz	150	3	18
2% milk	6 fl oz	165	5	27
Whole milk	6 fl oz	180	7	35

Coffee & Coffee Beverages
Black, regular

	AMOUNT	CALORIES	FAT GRAMS	% FAT
Brewed	6 fl oz	5	0	0
Instant, powdered	6 fl oz	5	0	0

Additions

	AMOUNT	CALORIES	FAT GRAMS	% FAT
Half-and-half	1 tbsp	20	2	90
Light table cream	1 tbsp	30	3	90
Milk				
Skim	1 tbsp	5	0	0
Whole	1 tbsp	10	.5	45

	AMOUNT	CALORIES	FAT-GRAMS	% FAT
Nondairy lightener				
Liquid	1 tbsp	20	2	90
Powdered	1 tsp	10	1	90
Sugar	1 tsp	15	0	0
	1 lump	15	0	0
	1 pkt	25	0	0
Sugar substitute	1 pkt	0-5	0	0
Café au lait	6 fl oz	60	3	30
Caffe con latte				
Small				
w/ skim milk	8 fl oz	60	.4	6
w/ whole milk	8 fl oz	100	5	45
Medium				
w/ skim milk	14 fl oz	110	.5	4
w/ whole milk	14 fl oz	180	10	50
Large				
w/ skim milk	16 fl oz	130	.5	4
w/ whole milk	16 fl oz	220	11	45
Cappuccino				
Small				
w/ skim milk	8 fl oz	40	.2	5
w/ whole milk	8 fl oz	70	4	51
Medium				
w/ skim milk	14 fl oz	60	.3	5
w/ whole milk	14 fl oz	110	6	49
Large				
w/ skim milk	16 fl oz	80	.4	5
w/ whole milk	16 fl oz	140	7	45
Espresso	3 fl oz	0	0	0

BEVERAGES

	AMOUNT	CALORIES	FAT-GRAMS	% FAT
Iced coffee				
w/ sugar and milk	8 fl oz	40	2	45
Irish coffee	9 fl oz	110	3	25
Mocha				
Small				
w/ skim milk	8 fl oz	150	8	48
w/ whole milk	8 fl oz	180	12	60
Medium				
w/ skim milk	14 fl oz	230	11	43
w/ whole milk	14 fl oz	290	18	56
Large				
w/ skim milk	16 fl oz	310	15	44
w/ whole milk	16 fl oz	390	25	58
Fruit Drinks				
Black cherry cooler	8 fl oz	90	0	0
Cranberry juice				
cocktail	6 fl oz	110	0	0
Fruit juice float	8 fl oz	205	7	30
Fruit punch	6 fl oz	85	0	0
Lemonade	8 fl oz	100	0	0
Limeade	8 fl oz	100	0	0
Fruit Juices				
Apple	6 fl oz	90	0	0
Apple cider	6 fl oz	90	0	0
Apple-cranberry	6 fl oz	85	0	0
Apple-raspberry	6 fl oz	100	0	0
Cherry	6 fl oz	100	0	0
Cranapple	6 fl oz	120	0	0

	AMOUNT	CALORIES	FAT-GRAMS	% FAT
Cranberry	6 fl oz	100	0	0
Cranberry-grape	6 fl oz	130	0	0
Grape	6 fl oz	110	0	0
Grapefruit	6 fl oz	70	0	0
Lemon	2 tbsp	10	0	0
Lime	2 tbsp	10	0	0
Orange	6 fl oz	90	0	0
Orange-grapefruit	6 fl oz	80	0	0
Orange-pineapple	6 fl oz	80	0	0
Peach	6 fl oz	100	0	0
Pineapple	6 fl oz	100	0	0
Pineapple-grapefruit	6 fl oz	90	0	0
Prune	6 fl oz	120	0	0
Milk				
Skim milk	8 fl oz	85	0	0
1% milk	8 fl oz	105	3	26
2% milk	8 fl oz	120	5	38
Whole milk	8 fl oz	150	8	48
Buttermilk	8 fl oz	100	2	18
Milk Drinks				
Chocolate milk, prepared w/				
Skim milk	8 fl oz	140	0	0
1% milk	8 fl oz	160	3	17
2% milk	8 fl oz	180	5	25
Whole milk	8 fl oz	210	8	34
Eggnog	8 fl oz	410	28	62
Eggnog, chocolate	8 fl oz	450	26	52

	AMOUNT	CALORIES	FAT-GRAMS	% FAT
Milk shake				
Chocolate	10 fl oz	360	11	28
Chocolate malt	10 fl oz	405	20	44
Strawberry	10 fl oz	320	8	23
Vanilla	10 fl oz	315	8	23
Strawberry-flavored				
milk	8 fl oz	210	8	34
Yogurt smoothie	8 fl oz	135	3	20
Tea				
Iced tea	8 fl oz	5	0	0
Iced tea drink				
Regular	16 fl oz	175	0	0
Diet	16 fl oz	10	0	0
Regular tea				
Bag	6 fl oz	0	0	0
Brewed	6 fl oz	0	0	0
Instant	6 fl oz	0	0	0
Instant, sugar-free	6 fl oz	0	0	0
Additions				
Half-and-half	1 tbsp	20	2	90
Honey	1 tsp	20	0	0
Lemon	1 pc	0	0	0
Milk				
Skim	1 tbsp	5	0	0
Whole	1 tbsp	10	.5	45
Nondairy lightener				
Liquid	1 tbsp	20	2	90
Powdered	1 tsp	10	1	90

	AMOUNT	CALORIES	FAT-GRAMS	% FAT
Sugar	1 tsp	15	0	0
	1 lump	15	0	0
	1 pkt	25	0	0
Sugar substitute	1 pkt	0-5	0	0
Russian tea	6 fl oz	100	0	0
Spiced tea	6 fl oz	100	0	0
Texas red-eye tea	6 fl oz	45	0	0
Vegetable Juices				
Carrot juice	6 fl oz	75	0	0
Tomato juice	6 fl oz	30	0	0
Tomato juice, spicy	6 fl oz	40	0	0
Vegetable juice cocktail	6 fl oz	35	0	0
Vegetable juice, spicy	6 fl oz	40	0	0

BREADS, CRACKERS & ROLLS

	AMOUNT	CALORIES	FAT-GRAMS	% FAT
Apple kuchen	1 serving	290	12	37
Apple streusel	1 slice	130	4	28
Bagels (3½"):				
Cinnamon & raisin bagel	1	195	1	5
Egg bagel	1	200	2	9
Oat bran bagel	1	150	1	6
Onion bagel	1	195	1	5
Plain bagel	1	195	1	5
Poppy seed bagel	1	195	1	5
Banana bread	1 slice	115	6	47
Biscuits:				
(*See* "Breakfast Foods" for biscuit with egg, biscuit with ham, etc.)				
Buttermilk biscuit (1 oz)	1	100	4	36
Cheese biscuit	1	230	11	43
Plain biscuit (1 oz)	1	100	4	36
Scone	1	365	14	33
Shortcake biscuit	1	300	16	48
Southern biscuit	1	195	8	37
Blueberry muffin (1.5 oz)	1	195	10	46
Bran muffin (1.5 oz)	1	125	6	33

	AMOUNT	CALORIES	FAT-GRAMS	% FAT
Breads:				
Banana bread	1 slice	115	6	47
Buttermilk bread	1 slice	75	2	24
Cheese bread	1 slice	180	10	50
Chorizo bread	1 slice	345	21	55
Country oat bread	1 slice	90	2	20
Corn bread (4" × 4")	1 serving	280	11	36
Cracked wheat bread	1 slice	70	2	26
Dark wheat bread	1 slice	80	1	11
Dill rye bread	1 slice	80	1	11
Egg bread	1 slice	115	2	16
English mead bread	1 slice	115	2	15
Focaccia	1 slice	175	6	31
Focaccia w/ vegetable topping & cheese	1 slice	295	12	37
French bread	1 slice	70	1	13
Garlic bread	1 slice	110	7	56
Green chili bread	1 slice	160	2	11
Grilled herb flatbread	1 slice	265	13	44
Honey wheat bread	1 slice	70	1	13
Irish soda bread	1 slice	145	2	12
Italian bread	1 slice	70	1	13
Italian bread w/ tomato, basil & mozzarella	1 slice	180	5	25
Italian bomba bread	1 wedge	360	12	30
Italian rosemary bread	1 slice	75	1	12
Multi-grain bread	1 slice	80	1	11
Navajo fry bread (5" diameter)	1 slice	300	9	27

	AMOUNT	CALORIES	FAT-GRAMS	% FAT
Oat-bran bread	1 slice	70	1	13
Oatmeal bread	1 slice	75	1	12
Pita bread (2 oz)	1 pocket	160	1	6
Pumpernickel	1 slice	80	1	11
Raisin bread	1 slice	70	1	13
Rye bread	1 slice	60	1	14
Seven-grain bread	1 slice	65	1	14
Sourdough bread	1 slice	70	1	13
Tenderfoot bread	1 slice	270	12	40
Vienna bread	1 slice	80	1	11
White bread	1 slice	80	1	11
Whole-wheat bread, 100% stone ground	1 slice	70	1	13
Bread spreads:				
Apple butter	1 tbsp	35	0	0
Apple jelly	1 tbsp	50	0	0
Butter (1 pat)	1 tsp	36	4	100
Grape jelly	1 tbsp	50	0	0
Honey	1 tbsp	65	0	0
Jam, all flavors	1 tbsp	50	0	0
Jam, sugar-free	1 tbsp	15	0	0
Jelly, all flavors	1 tbsp	50	0	0
Margarine (1 pat)	1 tsp	34	4	100
Whipped	1 tsp	70	7	100
Orange marmalade	1 tbsp	50	0	0
Peach butter	1 tbsp	35	0	0
Preserves, all flavors	1 tbsp	50	0	0
Bread sticks:				
Italian bread sticks	1 stick	45	1	19
Onion bread sticks	1 stick	40	1	23

	AMOUNT	CALORIES	FAT-GRAMS	% FAT
Plain bread sticks	1 stick	40	1	23
Sesame bread sticks	1 stick	50	2	36
Soft bread sticks	1 stick	70	2	26
Soft cheddar sticks	1 stick	100	6	53
Soft pretzels (1 oz each)	1 stick	125	2	14
Brioche	1 slice	135	5	33
Bruschetta w/ olives & tomatoes	1 slice	240	20	75
Buns:				
Chinese steamed bun	1 med	190	8	38
Hamburger bun (1.5 oz)	1	125	2	14
Hamburger bun (1.5 oz) reduced-calorie	1	85	1	11
Hot dog bun (1.5 oz)	1	120	2	15
Hot dog bun (1.5 oz), reduced-calorie	1	85	1	11
Kaiser bun	1 med	185	3	15
Butterhorn	1	330	18	49
Buttermilk biscuit (1 oz)	1	100	4	36
Cake-type doughnut				
Plain (1.5 oz)	1	165	8	44
Sugared (1.6 oz)	1	185	8	39
Cheese bread (1 slice bread, 1 oz cheese)	1 serving	180	10	50
Cheese crackers	14	70	4	51
Chocolate-covered doughnut	1	180	10	50

	AMOUNT	CALORIES	FAT-GRAMS	% FAT
Cinnamon roll	1	290	9	28
Coffee cake (2.2 oz)	1 slice	320	17	48
Corn bread (4" × 4")	1 serving	280	11	36
Corn fritter	1	60	2	29
Corn tortilla				
(6" diameter)	1	70	1	13
Cracked wheat crackers	4	110	4	33
Crackers:				
Cheese crackers	14	70	4	51
Chicken in a Biskit	7	70	4	51
Cracked wheat				
crackers	4	110	4	33
Crispbread crackers	3	60	2	30
Hearty wheat crackers	4	100	4	36
Lahvosh	1	30	1	30
Melba toast cracker	1	20	0	0
Milk crackers	1	55	2	33
Oyster crackers	16	60	2	30
Ritz crackers	4	70	4	51
Rye crisps	4	90	0	0
Saltines	2	25	1	36
Triscuits	7	145	5	31
Toasted sesame cracker	1	30	0	0
Water biscuit	3	90	3	30
Wheatsworth crackers	5	70	3	38
Wheat thins	7	80	4	45
Crepes (unfilled)	2	150	7	42
Danish pastry				
Almond (2.3 oz)	1	280	16	51
Apple (2.5 oz)	1	265	13	44

	AMOUNT	CALORIES	FAT-GRAMS	% FAT
Cheese (2.5 oz)	1	265	16	54
Cinnamon (2.3 oz)	1	260	15	52
Plain (2.5 oz)	1	220	12	49
Raisin (2.5 oz)	1	265	13	44
Raspberry (2.5 oz)	1	265	13	44
Strawberry (2.5 oz)	1	265	13	44
Dinner roll (1 oz)	1	120	2	15
Doughnuts:				
Cake-type doughnut				
Plain (1.5 oz)	1	165	8	44
Sugared (1.6 oz)	1	185	8	39
Chocolate-covered				
doughnut	1	180	10	50
Creme-filled doughnut				
(3 oz)	1	310	21	61
French cruller, glazed				
(1.5 oz)	1	170	8	42
Honey bun (2.1 oz)	1	240	14	53
Jelly-filled doughnut				
(2.3 oz)	1	225	9	36
Raised doughnut,				
plain	1	120	4	30
Sopapilla	1	170	7	37
Sugared doughnut				
(2.1 oz)	1	190	10	47
Yeast doughnut,				
glazed (2.1 oz)	1	240	14	53
English muffin	1	130	1	7
Focaccia	1 slice	175	6	31
French bread	1 slice	70	1	13

	AMOUNT	CALORIES	FAT-GRAMS	% FAT
French roll (1.3 oz)	1	140	2	13
French toast	2 slices	255	7	24
Fruit square	1	250	3	11
Garlic bread	1 slice	110	7	56
Green chili bread	1 slice	160	2	11
Gruyère puff ring	⅛ ring	205	13	57
Hamburger bun (1.5 oz)	1	125	2	14
Hamburger bun (1.5 oz), reduced-calorie	1	85	1	11
Hard roll (3½")	1	140	2	13
Hot dog bun (1.5 oz)	1	120	2	15
Hot dog bun (1.5 oz), reduced-calorie	1	85	1	11
Hush puppies (1.5 oz each)	2	140	5	32
Italian bread	1 slice	70	1	13
Italian bread sticks	1 stick	45	1	19
Jelly-filled doughnut (2.3 oz)	1	225	9	36
Melba toast (chef-prepared)				
Anchovy	1 slice	110	5	40
Cheese	1 slice	105	5	43
Garlic	1 slice	165	6	32
Herb	1 slice	165	6	32
Peanut butter	1 slice	110	5	40
Plain	1 slice	115	6	46
Sesame	1 slice	115	6	46

	AMOUNT	CALORIES	FAT-GRAMS	% FAT
Muffins:				
Regular size (1.5 oz)				
Apple	1	205	7	30
Blueberry	1	195	10	46
Bran	1	125	6	33
Bran raisin	1	190	6	28
Corn	1	180	7	35
Extra-large size (5 oz)				
Bran	1	405	21	44
Poppy	1	495	22	39
Onion bagel	1	195	1	5
Oyster crackers	16	60	2	30
Panettone	1 wedge	375	15	36
Panne	1 slice	110	4	32
Phyllo dough	1 oz	74	0	0
Pita bread (2 oz)	1 pocket	160	1	6
Pumpernickel bread	1 slice	80	1	11
Pizza bread (1 slice bread, 1 oz cheese)	1 serving	200	10	45
Plain bagel	1	195	1	5
Popovers	1.4 oz	100	4	37
Ritz crackers	4	70	4	51
Rolls:				
Brown 'n' serve roll (1 oz)	1	85	2	21
Butter corn roll	1 med	200	11	49
Cheese roll (2.3 oz)	1	240	12	45
Dinner roll (1 oz)	1	120	2	15
French roll (1.3 oz)	1	140	2	13
Hamburger roll (1.5 oz)	1	125	2	14

	AMOUNT	CALORIES	FAT-GRAMS	% FAT
Hamburger roll (1.5 oz), reduced-calorie	I	85	I	II
Hard roll (3½ inch)	I	140	2	13
Hot dog roll (1.5 oz)	I	120	2	15
Hot dog roll (1.5 oz), reduced-calorie	I	85	I	II
Onion roll (1.3 oz)	I	150	3	18
Parkerhouse (1 oz)	I oz	120	I	7
Sourdough roll (2.2 oz)	I	150	2	12
Submarine roll (4.7 oz)	I	155	2	33
Vienna roll (1 oz)	I	95	3	28
Wheat roll (1 oz)	I	75	2	24
Rye bread	I slice	60	I	14
Saltines	2	25	I	36
Scone	I	363	14	33
Sopapilla	I	170	10	33
Sourdough bread	I slice	70	I	13
Sourdough roll (2.2 oz)	I	150	2	12
Spoon bread	2 oz	155	6	35
Sticky bun	I	245	10	37
Sweet breads:				
Apple streusel	I slice	130	4	28
Banana nut bread	I slice	165	6	33
Boston brown bread (3¼ × ½")	I slice	95	I	10
Coffee cake (2.2 oz)	I slice	320	17	48
Cranberry bread	I slice	95	4	37
Danish krengle (2.2 oz)	I sq	230	14	55

	AMOUNT	CALORIES	FAT-GRAMS	% FAT
Danish pastry.				
See main entry.				
Danish twist	1	120	6	45
French crumb cake	1 slice	300	16	48
Fruit square	1	250	3	11
Pumpkin bread	1 slice	100	4	37
Sally Lunn	1 slice	240	11	41
Swedish limpa	1 slice	80	1	11
Sweet rolls/buns				
(medium-size):				
Butterhorn	1	330	18	49
Caramel bun	1	205	8	35
Caramel nut roll	1	230	11	43
Cinnamon roll	1	290	9	28
Fruit-filled roll	1	220	7	29
Hot cross bun	1	155	4	23
Orange roll	1	195	6	28
Santa Lucia bun	1	205	9	39
Sticky bun	1	245	10	37
Sweet potato bun	1	125	1	7
Sweet roll (2½ oz)	1	225	8	32
Tortilla				
Corn (6" diameter)	1	70	1	13
Flour (7" diameter)	1	85	2	21
White bread	1 slice	80	1	11
Whole-wheat bread,				
100% stone ground	1 slice	70	1	13
Pancakes (6")				
Banana pancakes	2	320	11	31
Blueberry pancakes	2	310	11	32

BREADS/CRACKERS/ROLLS

	AMOUNT	CALORIES	FAT-GRAMS	% FAT
Buckwheat pancakes	2	275	6	20
Buttermilk pancakes	2	330	10	27
Cherry pancakes	2	335	11	29
Corn meal pancakes	3	145	1	6
Johnnycakes	2	175	3	15
Plain pancakes	2	340	10	26

Pancake & waffle toppings:

	AMOUNT	CALORIES	FAT-GRAMS	% FAT
Butter	1 tbsp	100	1	100
	1 tsp/pat	35	4	100
Whipped	1 tbsp	60	7	100
Margarine				
Soft	1 tbsp	100	11	100
Stick	1 tbsp	100	11	100
	1 tsp/pat	35	4	100
Syrups				
Genovese	1 tbsp	50	0	0
Log Cabin Syrup	1 oz	100	0	0
Buttered	1 oz	105	0	0
Country Kitchen	1 oz	100	0	0
Lite	1 oz	60	0	0
Maple Honey	1 oz	105	0	0
Raspberry	1 tbsp	50	0	0
Strawberry	1 tbsp	50	0	0
Waffles				
Round (7" diameter)	1	280	19	61
Square (9")	1	600	40	60

Waffle toppings.
See Pancakes.

BREAKFAST FOODS

	AMOUNT	CALORIES	FAT-GRAMS	% FAT
Bacon				
Medium slice	2 strips	70	5	71
Thick slice	2 strips	100	8	72
Bacon, Canadian	2 slices	85	4	42
Bacon & Egg Breakfast				
(3 strips bacon, 2 fried				
eggs, 1 cup hash brown				
potatoes, 2 slices toast				
w/ margarine)	1 serving	900	54	54
Bagels (3½"):				
Cinnamon &				
raisin bagel	1	195	1	5
Egg bagel	1	200	2	9
Oat bran bagel	1	150	1	6
Onion bagel	1	195	1	5
Plain bagel	1	195	1	5
w/ 1 oz regular				
cream cheese	1	275	8	26
w/ 1 oz reduced-calorie				
cream cheese	1	255	6	21
w/ 1 oz fat-free				
cream cheese	1	220	1	4
Poppy seed bagel	1	195	1	5

	AMOUNT	CALORIES	FAT-GRAMS	% FAT
Belgian waffle w/ fruit &				
whipped topping	1 serving	900	32	31
w/ 2 oz ham	1 serving	1,000	35	31
w/ 2 strips bacon	1 serving	970	37	34
w/ 2 sausage links	1 serving	1,080	48	40
Biscuits:				
Biscuit & gravy	1 serving	275	14	46
Biscuits & Gravy				
Breakfast (2 biscuits,				
½ cup gravy, 2 eggs,				
2 sausage links, &				
2 strips bacon)	1 serving	1,110	65	53
Biscuit & sausage	1 serving	535	38	64
Biscuit, meat & gravy	1 serving	480	31	58
Biscuit w/ egg	1 serving	315	20	57
Biscuit w/ egg & bacon	1 serving	460	31	61
Biscuit w/ egg & sausage	1 serving	580	39	61
Biscuit w/ egg & steak	1 serving	425	28	53
Biscuit w/ egg, cheese				
& bacon	1 serving	480	31	58
Biscuit w/ ham	1 serving	390	18	42
Biscuit w/ sausage	1 serving	485	32	59
Biscuit w/ steak	1 serving	455	26	51
Buttermilk biscuit				
(1 oz)	1	100	4	36
Cheese biscuit (1 oz)	1	230	11	43
Plain biscuit (1 oz)	1	100	4	36
Scone	1	365	14	33
Shortcake biscuit	1	300	16	48
Southern biscuit	1	195	8	37

	AMOUNT	CALORIES	FAT-GRAMS	% FAT
Blintz, cheese	3	375	17	40
Breakfast cereals, cooked				
Cornmeal mush				
(cornmeal, butter)	1 cup	155	6	35
Cream of rice	¾ cup	110	0	0
Cream of wheat	¾ cup	110	0	0
Farina	⅔ cup	80	0	0
Corn grits	½ cup	55	0	0
Hominy quick grits				
(uncooked)	¼ cup	150	0	0
Oat bran	⅔ cup	110	1	8
Oatmeal	⅔ cup	110	1	8
Breakfast cereals,				
ready-to-eat				
All-Bran	⅔ cup	70	1	13
Alpha Bits	1 cup	110	0	0
Boo Berry	1 cup	110	0	0
Bran Flakes	⅔ cup	90	0	0
Cinnamon Toast Crunch	1 cup	120	3	22
Cheerios	1¼ cup	110	2	16
Chex	⅔ cup	90	0	0
Cocoa Puffs	1 cup	110	1	8
Corn Flakes	1 cup	100	0	0
Frankenberry	1 cup	110	1	8
Froot Loops	1 cup	110	0	0
Frosted Flakes	¾ cup	110	0	0
Fruit & Fibre	½ cup	90	0	0
Fruity Pebbles	1 cup	120	1	8
Granola	¼ cup	125	4	28
w/ raisins	¼ cup	125	4	29

BREAKFAST FOODS

	AMOUNT	CALORIES	FAT GRAMS	% FAT
Grape-Nuts	¼ cup	110	0	0
Flakes	⅞ cup	100	1	9
Honeycomb	1⅓ cup	110	1	8
Lucky Charms	1 cup	110	1	8
Muesli	½ cup	160	3	17
Mueslix Five Grain	½ cup	150	2	12
Nutri-Grain Wheat	⅔ cup	100	0	0
& Raisin	⅔ cup	130	0	0
Oat Bran Flakes	½ cup	100	0	0
Post Toasties	1¼ cup	108	0	0
Product 19	1 cup	100	0	0
Puffed Rice	1 cup	40	0	0
Raisin Bran	¾ cup	120	1	7
Rice Krispies	1 cup	110	0	0
Shredded Wheat	1 biscuit	85	0	0
Bite Size	⅔ cup	110	1	8
Special K	1 cup	110	0	0
Sugar Frosted Flakes	¾ cup	110	0	0
Total	1 cup	110	1	8
Total Corn Flakes	1 cup	110	1	8
Trix	1 cup	110	1	8
Wheaties	1 cup	110	1	8

With Milk

If milk is added, fat and
calories increase as follows:

	AMOUNT	CALORIES	FAT GRAMS	% FAT
Skim milk	4 fl oz	45	0	0
	8 fl oz	85	0	0
2% milk	4 fl oz	60	3	38
	8 fl oz	120	5	3

	AMOUNT	CALORIES	FAT GRAMS	% FAT
Whole milk	4 fl oz	80	4	48
	8 fl oz	150	8	48
Coffee & coffee beverages				
Black, regular				
Brewed	6 fl oz	5	0	0
Instant, powdered	6 fl oz	5	0	0
Additions				
Half-and-half	1 tbsp	20	2	90
Light table cream	1 tbsp	30	3	90
Milk				
Skim	1 tbsp	5	0	0
Whole	1 tbsp	10	.5	45
Nondairy lightener				
Liquid	1 tbsp	20	2	90
Powdered	1 tsp	10	1	90
Sugar	1 tsp	15	0	0
	1 lump	15	0	0
	1 pkt	25	0	0
Sugar substitute	1 pkt	0-5	0	0
Café au lait	6 fl oz	60	3	30
Caffe con latte				
Small				
w/ skim milk	8 fl oz	60	.4	6
w/ whole milk	8 fl oz	100	5	45
Medium				
w/ skim milk	14 fl oz	110	.5	4
w/ whole milk	14 fl oz	180	10	50
Large				
w/ skim milk	16 fl oz	130	.5	4
w/ whole milk	16 fl oz	220	11	45

	AMOUNT	CALORIES	FAT-GRAMS	% FAT
Cappuccino				
Small				
w/ skim milk	8 fl oz	40	.2	5
w/ whole milk	8 fl oz	70	4	51
Medium				
w/ skim milk	14 fl oz	60	.3	5
w/ whole milk	14 fl oz	110	6	49
Large				
w/ skim milk	16 fl oz	80	.4	5
w/ whole milk	16 fl oz	140	7	45
Espresso	3 fl oz	0	0	0
Mocha				
Small				
w/ skim milk	8 fl oz	150	8	48
w/ whole milk	8 fl oz	180	12	60
Medium				
w/ skim milk	14 fl oz	230	11	43
w/ whole milk	14 fl oz	290	18	56
Large				
w/ skim milk	16 fl oz	310	15	44
w/ whole milk	16 fl oz	390	25	58
Cocoa & hot chocolate				
Prepared w/ water	6 fl oz	50	0	0
Diet	6 fl oz	20	0	0
Prepared w/				
Skim milk	6 fl oz	135	2	10
1% milk	6 fl oz	150	3	18
2% milk	6 fl oz	65	5	27
Whole milk	6 fl oz	180	7	35

	AMOUNT	CALORIES	FAT-GRAMS	% FAT
Crepes (unfilled)	2	150	7	42
Croissant (2 oz)	1	235	12	46
Apple	1	145	5	31
Cheese	1	235	12	46
Doughnuts:				
Cake-type doughnut				
Plain (1.5 oz)	1	165	8	44
Sugared (1.6 oz)	1	185	8	39
Chocolate-covered				
doughnut	1	180	8	50
Creme-filled doughnut				
(3 oz)	1	310	21	61
French cruller,				
glazed (1.5 oz)	1	170	8	42
Honey bun (2.1 oz)	1	240	14	53
Jelly-filled doughnut				
(2.3 oz)	1	225	9	36
Raised doughnut	1	120	4	30
Sopapilla	1	170	7	37
Sugared doughnut				
(1.6 oz)	1	190	10	47
Yeast doughnut, glazed				
(2.1 oz)	1	240	14	53
Eggs:				
Bacon & Egg Breakfast (3 strips bacon, 2 fried eggs, 1 cup hash brown potatoes, 2 slices toast w/ margarine)	1 serving	900	54	54

	AMOUNT	CALORIES	FAT-GRAMS	% FAT
Baked (shirred) eggs w/ cheese	2 eggs	265	22	74
Boiled egg	1	75	5	41
Breakfast pizza (eggs, olive, mushrooms, tomatoes)	⅙ of 12" pie	325	21	58
Calf brains & eggs	1 serving	690	57	75
Canadian Bacon & Egg Breakfast (2 slices Canadian bacon, 2 fried eggs, 1 cup hash brown potatoes, 2 slices toast w/ margarine)	1 serving	775	43	50
Cheesy egg roll-up tortilla	1	395	24	55
Egg blintzes	2	185	6	29
Egg substitute, scrambled	2 eggs	130	6	43
Egg turnover w/ cheese sauce	1 serving	470	34	65
Eggs à la goldenrod (eggs, toast, cream sauce)	5 oz	810	52	58
Eggs à la king	5 oz	690	43	56
Eggs à la Purgatory	2 eggs	220	14	57
Eggs w/ avocado sauce	2 eggs	400	33	74
Eggs Benedict (½ English muffin, 1 egg, ham, sauce)	1 serving	410	32	70

	AMOUNT	CALORIES	FAT-GRAMS	% FAT
Eggs Benedict casserole	1 serving	395	28	64
Eggs w/ black beans & plantains	2 eggs	400	33	74
Eggs in cheese sauce	6 oz	355	22	56
Eggs on English muffin	2 eggs	280	17	55
Eggs Florentine	2 tarts	530	40	68
Eggs Park Avenue (eggs, lox, sour cream, cream cheese, Hollandaise sauce)	6 oz	935	92	88
Eggs Romano (2 eggs, spinach, olives, Romano)	1 serving	375	25	60
Eggs in shirts	3 eggs	440	40	82
Eggs Sojourn (2 eggs, crab & shrimp meat, English muffin, Hollandaise sauce)	1 serving	1,790	159	80
Egg on tortilla (1 egg, 1 corn tortilla, cheese, salsa)	1 serving	345	25	65
Fried egg	1	105	8	69
Fried Egg Breakfast (2 eggs)				
w/ 1 cup hash brown potatoes & 2 slices plain toast	1 serving	560	29	47
w/ 1 cup hash brown potatoes, 3 oz ham, & 2 slices plain toast	1 serving	760	35	41

BREAKFAST FOODS

	AMOUNT	CALORIES	FAT-GRAMS	% FAT
w/ 1 cup hash brown potatoes & 2 slices toast w/ margarine	1 serving	690	39	51
w/ 1 cup hash brown potatoes, 3 strips bacon, 2 slices toast w/ margarine	1 serving	795	47	53
w/ 2 pancakes w/ syrup & margarine, 2 sausage links & 2 strips bacon	1 serving	1,050	52	43
w/ 1 cup hash brown potatoes, 4 sausage links & 2 slices toast w/ margarine	1 serving	1,040	70	61
w/ 3 pancakes w/ syrup & margarine, 3 sausage links & 3 strips bacon	1 serving	1,490	76	46
Frittata (3 eggs) w/ mushrooms	1 serving	310	23	67
w/ zucchini, cheese & artichokes	1 serving	585	47	72
Ham & Egg Breakfast (2 fried eggs, 1 cup hash brown potatoes, 3 oz ham & 2 slices toast w/ margarine)	1 serving	760	35	41
w/ 3 pancakes w/ syrup & margarine	1 serving	1,530	57	34

	AMOUNT	CALORIES	FAT-GRAMS	% FAT
Huevos con queso in tortilla (2 eggs, cheese tortilla sauce)	1 serving	745	53	64
Huevos leone (bacon omelet w/ tortilla)	1 serving	565	42	67
Huevos rancheros	1 serving	390	25	58
Hungarian gulyas (egg, yogurt, ham, cheese, sunflower seeds)	1 serving	425	34	72
Oeufs Antoine (eggs, bacon, capers, English muffin, Mornay sauce)	1 serving	705	50	64
Omelets (3 eggs)				
Bacon omelet	1	375	28	67
Basque omelet (w/ peppers, onion, tomato)	1	430	36	75
Cheese omelet	1	355	26	66
Cheese Omelet Breakfast (1 cup hash brown potatoes, 3 strips bacon, 2 slices toast w/ margarine)	1 serving	940	57	55
w/ 3 pancakes w/ syrup & margarine	1 serving	1,710	79	42

	AMOUNT	CALORIES	FAT-GRAMS	% FAT
Farmer-style omelet (eggs, onion, ham, potatoes)	1	405	30	67
Ham omelet	1	295	21	64
Mushroom omelet	1	300	22	66
Plain omelet	1	330	21	57
Spanish omelet (w/ Creole sauce)	1	350	25	64
Western omelet (eggs, bacon, ham, onion, peppers)	1	355	25	63
Poached egg	1	75	5	41
Creamy poached egg (1 egg on ½ English muffin w/ cheese sauce)	1 serving	325	20	56
Poached eggs Henri (eggs, toast, Canadian bacon, asparagus, Hollandaise sauce)	1 serving	690	55	72
Sausage and Egg Breakfast (2 fried eggs, 4 links sausage, 1 cup hash brown potatoes, 2 slices toast w/ margarine)	1 serving	1,030	71	62
w/ 3 pancakes w/ syrup & margarine	1 serving	1,750	83	43
Scrambled eggs (2 large eggs)	1 serving	200	15	68

	AMOUNT	CALORIES	FAT-GRAMS	% FAT
w/ 2 oz ham	1 serving	275	21	68
w/ herbs	1 serving	205	15	66
w/ mushrooms	1 serving	210	15	64
w/ smoked salmon	1 serving	305	19	56
Scrambled Egg Breakfast (2 large eggs)				
w/ 1 cup hash brown potatoes & 2 slices plain toast	1 serving	640	26	37
w/ 1 cup hash brown potatoes, 2 oz ham 2 slices plain toast	1 serving	740	29	35
w/ 1 cup hash brown potatoes & 2 slices toast w/ margarine	1 serving	770	36	42
w/ 1 cup hash brown potatoes, 3 strips bacon 2 slices toast w/ margarine	1 serving	875	44	45
w/ 2 pancakes w/ syrup & margarine, 2 sausage links & 2 strips bacon	1 serving	1,130	49	39
w/ 1 cup hash brown potatoes, 4 sausage links & 2 slices toast w/ margarine	1 serving	1,120	67	54
w/ 3 pancakes w/ syrup & margarine, 3 sausage links & 3 strips bacon	1 serving	1,570	73	42

	AMOUNT	CALORIES	FAT-GRAMS	% FAT
Scrambled egg substitute				
(= 2 eggs)	1 serving	130	6	43
w/ 1 cup hash brown potatoes & 2 slices plain toast	1 serving	480	18	35
w/ 1 cup hash brown potatoes, 2 oz ham, & 2 slices plain toast	1 serving	580	22	34
Scotch egg	1 serving	300	21	63
Soufflé (6 oz)				
Cheese	1 serving	325	24	66
Spinach	1 serving	320	18	51
Swiss eggs				
(3 eggs, Swiss cheese, Gruyère)	1 serving	505	44	78
Zucchini & egg crepes	2 crepes	445	29	58
English muffin	1	130	1	7
w/ jam (2 tsp)	1 serving	155	1	6
w/ 1 pat butter or margarine	1 serving	165	5	27
& jam (2 tsp)	1 serving	185	5	24
w/ cheese & sausage	1 serving	395	24	55
w/ egg, cheese & bacon	1 serving	490	31	57
w/ egg, cheese & Canadian bacon	1 serving	385	20	47
French toast (3 slices)				
w/ syrup only	1 serving	800	26	30
w/ 2 oz ham	1 serving	900	30	30

	AMOUNT	CALORIES	FAT-GRAMS	% FAT
w/ 2 strips bacon	I serving	870	32	33
w/ 2 sausage links	I serving	970	42	39
w/ syrup & margarine	I serving	910	33	33
w/ 2 oz ham	I serving	1,010	37	33
w/ 4 strips bacon	I serving	1,050	44	38
w/ 4 sausage links	I serving	1,260	65	47
Fruit juices				
Apple	6 fl oz	90	0	0
Apple cider	6 fl oz	90	0	0
Apple-cranberry	6 fl oz	85	0	0
Apple-raspberry	6 fl oz	100	0	0
Cherry	6 fl oz	100	0	0
Cranapple	6 fl oz	120	0	0
Cranberry	6 fl oz	100	0	0
Cranberry-grape	6 fl oz	130	0	0
Grape	6 fl oz	110	0	0
Grapefruit	6 fl oz	70	0	0
Orange	6 fl oz	90	0	0
Orange-grapefruit	6 fl oz	80	0	0
Orange-pineapple	6 fl oz	80	0	0
Peach	6 fl oz	100	0	0
Pineapple	6 fl oz	100	0	0
Pineapple-grapefruit	6 fl oz	90	0	0
Prune	6 fl oz	120	0	0
Ham, fried	2 oz	100	3	32
	3.5 oz	175	6	32
Muffins:				
Regular size (1.5 oz)				
Apple	I	205	7	30
Blueberry	I	195	10	46

	AMOUNT	CALORIES	FAT GRAMS	% FAT
Bran	1	125	6	33
Bran raisin	1	190	6	28
Corn	1	180	7	35
Extra-large size (5 oz)				
Bran	1	405	21	44
Poppy	1	495	22	39
Pancakes (6")				
Banana pancakes	2	320	11	31
Blueberry pancakes	2	310	11	32
Buckwheat pancakes	2	275	6	20
Buttermilk pancakes	2	330	10	27
Cherry pancakes	2	335	11	29
Cornmeal pancakes	3	145	1	6
Johnnycakes	2	175	3	15
Plain pancakes	2	340	10	26
Pancake & waffle toppings:				
Butter	1 tbsp	100	1	100
	1 tsp/pat	35	4	100
Whipped	1 tbsp	60	7	100
Margarine				
Soft	1 tbsp	100	11	100
Stick	1 tbsp	100	11	100
	1 tsp/pat	35	4	100
Syrups				
Genovese	1 tbsp	50	0	0
Log Cabin Syrup	1 oz	100	0	0
Buttered	1 oz	105	0	0
Country Kitchen	1 oz	100	0	0
Lite	1 oz	60	0	0

	AMOUNT	CALORIES	FAT-GRAMS	% FAT
Maple Honey	1 oz	105	0	0
Raspberry	1 tbsp	50	0	0
Strawberry	1 tbsp	50	0	0
Pancake Breakfast				
(4 pancakes)				
w/ syrup only	1 serving	870	16	17
w/ 2 oz ham	1 serving	970	20	18
w/ 2 strips bacon	1 serving	940	22	21
w/ 2 links sausage	1 serving	1,040	32	28
w/ syrup & margarine	1 serving	940	29	28
w/ 2 oz ham	1 serving	1,040	33	28
w/ 2 strips bacon	1 serving	1,080	40	33
w/ 2 links sausage	1 serving	1,290	62	43
Potatoes:				
Cottage fried potatoes	1 cup	370	14	34
Hash brown potatoes	1 cup	220	11	43
Home-fried potatoes	1 cup	440	16	33
Potatoes O'Brien	1 cup	330	14	38
Sausage				
Links	2	170	16	84
	4	340	32	84
Patty (3 oz)	1	330	33	90
Sweet breads:				
Apple streusel	1 slice	130	4	28
Banana nut bread	1 slice	165	6	33
Boston brown bread				
(3¼ × ½)	1 slice	95	1	10
Coffee cake	2½ oz	320	17	48
Cranberry bread	1 slice	95	4	37
Danish krengle	1 sq	230	14	55

	AMOUNT	CALORIES	FAT-GRAMS	% FAT
Danish pastry				
Almond (2.3 oz)	1	280	16	51
Apple (2.5 oz)	1	265	13	44
Cheese (2.5 oz)	1	265	16	54
Cinnamon (2.3 oz)	1	260	15	52
Plain	1	220	12	49
Raisin (2.5 oz)	1	265	13	44
Raspberry (2.5 oz)	1	265	13	44
Strawberry (2.5 oz)	1	265	13	44
Danish twist	1	120	6	45
French crumb cake	1 slice	300	16	48
Fruit square	1	250	3	11
Pumpkin bread	1 slice	100	4	37
Sally Lunn	1 slice	240	11	41
Swedish limpa	1 slice	80	1	11
Sweet rolls/buns:				
Butterhorn	1	330	18	49
Caramel bun	1	205	8	35
Caramel nut roll	1	230	11	43
Cinnamon roll	1	290	9	28
Fruit-filled roll	1	220	7	29
Hot cross bun	1	155	4	23
Orange roll	1	195	6	28
Santa Lucia bun	1	205	9	39
Sticky bun	1	245	10	37
Sweet potato bun	1	125	1	7
Sweet roll (2.5 oz)	1	225	8	32
Tea:				
Regular tea				
Bag	6 fl oz	0	0	0

	AMOUNT	CALORIES	FAT-GRAMS	% FAT
Brewed	6 fl oz	0	0	0
Instant	6 fl oz	0	0	0
Instant, sugar-free	6 fl oz	0	0	0
Additions				
Half-and-half	1 tbsp	20	2	90
Honey	1 tsp	20	0	0
Lemon	1 pc	0	0	0
Milk				
Skim	1 tbsp	5	0	0
Whole	1 tbsp	10	.5	45
Nondairy lightener				
Liquid	1 tbsp	20	2	90
Powdered	1 tsp	10	1	90
Sugar	1 tsp	15	0	0
	1 lump	15	0	0
	1 pkt	25	0	0
Sugar substitute	1 pkt	0–5	0	0
Russian tea	6 fl oz	100	0	0
Spiced tea	6 fl oz	100	0	0
Texas red-eye tea	6 fl oz	45	0	0
Waffles				
Round (7" diameter)	1	280	19	61
Square (9" diameter)	1	600	40	60
Waffle toppings. *See* Pancakes.				
Yogurt (8 oz)				
Plain				
Nonfat	1 serving	125	0	0
Low-fat	1 serving	145	4	25
Fruit, low-fat	1 serving	225	3	12
Vanilla, low-fat	1 serving	195	3	14

BREAKFAST FOODS

CHEESE & CHEESE DISHES

	AMOUNT	CALORIES	FAT-GRAMS	% FAT
Asparagus w/ rarebit sauce	6 oz	525	34	58
Cheese:				
American	1 oz	90	7	70
Low-fat	1 oz	70	4	40
Fat-free	1 oz	45	0	0
Blue	1 oz	100	9	81
Bonbel	1 oz	100	8	72
Brie	1 oz	95	8	76
Cajun	1 oz	110	9	74
Camembert	1 oz	85	7	74
Cheddar	1 oz	110	9	74
Low-fat	1 oz	90	5	50
Fat-free	1 oz	45	0	0
Cottage cheese, creamed				
Full-fat	½ cup	120	5	37
Low-fat	½ cup	90	1	10
Cream cheese	1 oz	100	10	90
Light	1 oz	60	5	75
Fat-free	1 oz	25	0	0
Whipped	1 oz	100	10	90
Edam	1 oz	100	8	72

	AMOUNT	CALORIES	FAT-GRAMS	% FAT
Feta	1 oz	75	6	72
Gorgonzola	1 oz	100	8	72
Gouda	1 oz	110	9	74
Gruyère	1 oz	120	9	68
Havarti	1 oz	120	11	84
Jarlsberg	1 oz	100	7	63
Monterey Jack	1 oz	80	4	45
Mozzarella, low-moisture				
Whole-milk	1 oz	90	7	70
Part-skim	1 oz	80	5	56
Mozzarella, part-skim	1 oz	70	5	62
Nacho	1 oz	105	9	76
Parmesan, grated	1 tbsp	25	2	78
Port du Salut	1 oz	100	8	72
Pot cheese	1 oz	109	5	41
Provolone	1 oz	100	7	63
Ricotta				
Whole-milk	1 oz	60	5	75
Part-skim	1 oz	40	3	68
Fat-free	1 oz	25	0	0
Roquefort	1 oz	105	9	77
String cheese	1 oz	80	5	57
Swiss	1 oz	100	8	72
Taco, shredded	1 oz	100	9	81
Tilsit	1 oz	95	7	66
Cheese & bean enchilada	1	345	16	42
Cheese & beef enchilada	1	325	18	49
Cheese blintzes	3	375	17	40
Cinnamon	3	375	17	40

	AMOUNT	CALORIES	FAT-GRAMS	% FAT
Crabmeat	3	390	17	39
Pineapple	3	385	17	40
Shrimp	3	390	17	39
Cheeseburger				
(w/o mayo or				
mayo-type dressing)	1	320	15	42
Double	1	545	28	46
Extra-large	1	610	33	49
Cheesecake	⅛ of 9"cake	425	29	61
Cheese cubes (1 oz each)	3	330	27	74
Cheese dip	2 tbsp	50	4	72
Cheese enchilada	1	325	18	49
Cheese fries	1 cup	595	38	57
w/ ranch dressing	2 tbsp	750	54	66
Cheese fritters	3	365	16	40
Cheese omelet	1	355	26	66
Cheese pie	⅛ of 9"pie	330	17	46
Cheese pizza, 12"	1 pie	875	20	21
	⅛ pie	110	3	24
Cheese sauce	2 oz	105	8	68
Cheese soup made				
w/ milk	1 cup	230	15	59
Cheese spaetzle	8 oz	940	51	49
Cheese soufflé	5 oz	325	24	66
Cheese strata	6 oz	315	18	51
Chile relleno	1	340	24	64
Cream cheese brownies	2	390	23	53
Cream cheese pie	1 slice	385	25	58
Baked potato w/ cheese	1	475	29	54
& bacon	1	450	26	52

	AMOUNT	CALORIES	FAT-GRAMS	% FAT
Bean & cheese burrito	2	380	12	28
Emmentaler flan	⅙ of 9" pie	830	58	63
Fondue:				
Fontina (Italian)	6 oz	510	46	81
Swiss fondue w/ bread	1 serving	1,515	59	35
Frijoles w/ cheese	1 cup	225	8	31
Grilled cheese sandwich	1	360	23	57
w/ bacon	1	450	30	60
w/ chili	1	405	25	55
w/ ham	1	410	25	55
w/ olive	1	380	24	57
w/ tomato	1	370	23	56
Ham & cheese melt on hamburger bun	1	320	17	48
Hot provolone sandwich	1	380	18	43
Nachos w/ cheese	6–8	345	19	49
w/ beef & bean	6–8	570	30	49
Paschel pie (cheese, sausage, eggs)	⅙ of 10" pie	1,110	82	66
Polenta cheese torta	8 oz	560	28	45
Quiche (⅙ of 9" pie)				
Quiche Jambon Chardonnay	1 slice	1,075	74	62
Quiche Lorraine	1 slice	875	61	63
Quiche Suisse	1 slice	990	72	65
Ricotta quiche	1 slice	925	63	61
Seafood quiche	1 slice	1,005	67	60

	AMOUNT	CALORIES	FAT-GRAMS	% FAT
Rarebit:				
Asparagus w/ rarebit sauce	6 oz	525	34	58
Bacon rarebit	6 oz	585	41	63
Ham rarebit	6 oz	575	39	61
Onion rarebit (Swiss)	2 slices	945	65	62
Pineapple rarebit	6 oz	525	34	58
Rarebit in oven (Bavarian)	2 slices	620	26	38
Tomato rarebit	6 oz	530	35	59
Welsh rarebit	6 oz	500	34	61
Sbrinz casserole (Swiss)	8 oz	305	18	53
Shepherd's Yodel (Bavarian)	2 slices	800	55	62
Swiss bread rosti	6 oz	500	28	50
Swiss ramekin	8 oz	595	31	47
Tostada				
Bean & cheese	1	225	10	40
Beef & cheese	1	315	16	46
Welsh rarebit	6 oz	500	34	61

DESSERTS & TOPPINGS

	AMOUNT	CALORIES	FAT-GRAMS	% FAT
Almond torte	⅒ of 9" torte	280	20	64
Baklava (2" × 2")	1	430	29	61
Bars:				
Almond toffee bars	2	165	10	54
Chinese chews	2	395	16	37
French lemon bars	2	120	4	29
French nut loaf	1	390	25	57
Fudge nut loaf	1	390	18	41
Hermits	2	275	11	36
Magic Bars	2	205	12	53
Mincemeat strips	2	140	7	45
Orange-date bars	2	205	7	30
Peanut butter crunch	1 pc	235	9	34
Bavarians:				
Banana-lemon	4 oz	160	7	39
Caramel	4 oz	200	11	50
Chocolate	4 oz	245	13	48
Coffee	4 oz	220	15	62
Fruit-nut	4 oz	245	16	59
Orange cream	4 oz	170	7	37
Pineapple	4 oz	200	11	49

	AMOUNT	CALORIES	FAT-GRAMS	% FAT
Raspberry	4 oz	135	7	46
Strawberry	4 oz	150	7	42
Biscuit tortoni	3 oz	345	29	75
Blintzes:				
Cheese	3	375	17	40
Cherry	1	385	17	40
Cinnamon cheese	3	375	17	40
Pineapple cheese	3	385	17	40
Brownies:				
Bavarian brownie drop	1	125	8	58
Brownies				
Cake type	2	155	8	47
Chewy type	2	160	9	50
Butterscotch brownies	2	145	7	44
Chocolate coconut				
brownie	1	345	18	47
Cream cheese brownies	2	390	23	53
Cake:				
Angel food cake	1 slice	145	0	0
w/ icing		220	3	12
Applesauce cake	1 slice	245	9	33
Apricot upside-down				
cake	1 slice	245	9	33
Baked Alaska	5 oz	390	9	21
Banana cake	1 slice	260	9	31
w/ icing		335	12	32
Black Forest cake				
w/ icing	1 slice	530	20	34
Boston cream pie cake	1/12 of			
	10" cake	260	8	28

	AMOUNT	CALORIES	FAT-GRAMS	% FAT
Burnt sugar cake	1 slice	225	9	36
Butter rum pound cake	1/12 of			
	10" cake	480	19	36
Cannoli cake	1/12 of			
	9" cake	785	35	40
Carrot cake w/ cream cheese icing	1/16 of			
	10" cake	385	21	49
Carrot spice cake	1 slice	220	10	41
w/ icing		295	13	40
Cheesecake	1/8 of			
	9" cake	410	31	68
Chocolate	1/8 of			
	9" cake	425	29	61
Chocolate hazelnut	1/7 of			
	7" cake	400	32	72
Chocolate ricotta	1/8 of			
	8" cake	435	26	53
Peanut butter	1/8 of			
	9" cake	410	23	50
Pumpkin	1/8 of			
	9" cake	465	34	66
Strawberry	1/8 of			
	9" cake	530	31	53
Cherry jubilee cake	1 slice	130	7	49
Chiffon cake	1/12 of			
	10" cake	230	10	39
w/ icing		305	13	39
Chocolate cake roll	1 slice	360	11	27
w/ icing		465	19	37

	AMOUNT	CALORIES	FAT-GRAMS	% FAT
Chocolate chiffon cake	1/12 of 10" cake	235	10	38
w/ icing		335	17	45
Chocolate whipped cream cake	1/12 of 10" cake	400	22	49
Christmas fruitcake	1/32 of loaf	275	8	26
Devil's food cake	1 slice	190	8	38
w/ icing		295	15	46
Dutch apple cake	1 pc	220	7	29
English plum pudding	1 slice	270	7	23
French crumb cake	1 slice	365	16	39
Fruit coffee cake	1 slice	275	10	33
Fruit pudding cake	2.5 oz	195	7	32
Fruit whipped cream cake	1 slice	305	18	53
German chocolate cake	1 slice	225	12	48
w/ icing		330	19	52
Gingerbread	1 slice	200	8	36
Honeycomb crunch cake	1 slice	405	24	54
Lady Baltimore cake	1 slice	265	11	38
Nut torte	1 slice	195	10	47
Orange coffee cake	1 slice	185	6	29
Peach downside-up cake	1 slice	265	11	37
Peanut butter cake	1 slice	230	10	39
w/ icing		335	13	35
Pineapple upside-down cake	1 slice	255	10	35

	AMOUNT	CALORIES	FAT-GRAMS	% FAT
Plain cake	I slice	190	7	33
w/ buttercream icing		265	10	34
w/ chocolate icing		290	14	43
Poor man's cake	I slice	235	4	15
Pound cake	⅑ of			
	9" cake	365	21	52
Praline cake	I slice	310	19	55
Prune spice cake	I slice	200	8	36
Pumpkin cake	I slice	275	9	30
Sally Lunn	I slice	240	11	41
Spice cake	I slice	205	8	35
w/ icing		280	11	36
Sponge cake	I indiv cake	190	3	14
Sponge roll	I slice	125	2	14
Swiss nut cake	I slice	390	24	55
White cake	I slice	230	9	35
w/ icing		305	12	35
Cannoli	⅟₁₁ of			
	11" shell	530	35	60
Cassata	I slice	605	19	28
Chocolate éclair				
(2" × 4")	I	239	13	51
Chocolate pot de crème	4 oz	315	20	57
Cookies:				
Apricot strips	I	210	9	22
Biscotti (Italian cookies)	I	127	7	50
Brown sugar cookie	I	135	7	47
Butterscotch cookie	I	60	3	45
Cherry Winks	I	95	4	38
Chocolate candy cookie	I	120	4	30

	AMOUNT	CALORIES	FAT-GRAMS	% FAT
Chocolate-chip cookie	1	105	5	42
Chocolate crumb cookie	1	85	4	42
Chocolate drop cookie	1	165	6	33
Coconut-chip cookie	1	135	8	52
Coconut lace cookie	1	45	2	38
Crescent	1	100	7	64
Fortune cookie	1	65	4	55
Ginger cookie	1	165	5	28
Ginger crisp	1	60	2	29
Lady finger	1	40	1	20
Lebkuchen	1	55	1	16
Madeleines	2	85	5	53
Meringue cookie	1	35	0	0
Molasses cookie	1	155	7	40
Oatmeal cookie	1	160	7	39
Oatmeal raisin cookie	1	145	7	43
Oatmeal spice cookie	1	110	6	48
Peanut butter candy	1	125	6	43
Peanut butter cup	1	155	9	53
Raisin drop cookie	1	100	4	36
Refrigerator cookie	1	70	3	39
Sandtart	1	80	5	58
Shortbread	1	155	9	52
Snickerdoodle	1	80	3	35
Spritz	1	70	4	50
Sugar cookie	1	150	6	36
Sugar plum cookie	1	45	2	40
Swedish ginger cookie	1	40	2	43

	AMOUNT	CALORIES	FAT-GRAMS	% FAT
Turtle cookies	2	195	10	46
Vanilla butter cookies	2	65	3	42
Cream puff w/ custard				
filling (3½" × 2")	1	303	18	54
Crepes				
Crepes Suzette	3	600	31	46
Dessert crepe				
(unfilled)	1	135	7	47
Raspberry crepes	2	540	21	35
Custards:				
Burnt cream	4 oz	325	25	69
Caramel flan	¾ cup	230	6	23
Crème brulée	4 oz	325	25	69
Custard	4 oz	160	5	28
Spanish cream	4 oz	185	9	44
English trifle	4 oz	465	23	44
Fruit				
Apples				
Applesauce	1 cup	190	1	5
Baked apple	1	185	1	5
Baked date-nut apple	1	290	7	22
Caramel apple	1	430	20	42
Caramel fried apples	⅓ apple	205	5	22
Taffy apple	1	390	11	25
Apricot tart	⅛ of			
	10" pie	470	13	25
Apricots, stewed	6 halves	60	0	0
Banana dessert fritters	2	310	5	14
Cherries Jubilee				
(sauce only)	4 oz	65	0	0

	AMOUNT	CALORIES	FAT-GRAMS	% FAT
Cherry blintz	1	385	17	40
Fruit & 2 oz cheese	1 serving	310	18	52
Fruit compote	1 serving	90	0	0
Fruit cup	½ cup	55	0	0
Fruit-nut Bavarian	4 oz	245	16	59
Fruit plate (fruit only)	1 serving	80	0	0
Italian cream				
w/ raspberries	1 serving	265	16	55
Peaches flambé	4 oz	420	17	36
Pineapple cheese blintz	3	385	17	40
Poached pear				
w/ raspberry sauce	1 pear	490	12	22
Prunes, stewed	3 prunes	85	0	0
Prune whip	2 oz	130	1	7
Strawberries Romanoff	4 oz	115	4	31
Gelatin, all flavors	½ cup	80	0	0
Sugar-free	½ cup	10	0	0
Ice cream				
Fat-free, avg	½ cup	90	0	0
Sealtest Black Cherry	½ cup	100	0	0
Simple Pleasures				
Chocolate	½ cup	130	0	0
Low-fat (1%), avg	½ cup	80	1	11
Dreyer's Chocolate	½ cup	80	1	11
Healthy Choice				
Butter Pecan	½ cup	120	2	15
Premium (10%), avg	½ cup	135	7	47
Borden Chocolate	½ cup	160	10	56
Breyers Strawberry	½ cup	130	6	42
Dreyer's Vanilla	½ cup	160	10	56

	AMOUNT	CALORIES	FAT-GRAMS	% FAT
Super premium				
(16%), avg	½ cup	175	12	62
Ben & Jerry's				
Chocolate	½ cup	290	18	56
Häagen-Dazs				
Strawberry	½ cup	250	15	54
Vanilla	½ cup	260	17	57
Ice cream, soft-serve	½ cup	200	12	54
Ice cream bar,				
chocolate-coated:				
Premium, avg	1	180	12	60
Dolly Madison	1	200	12	54
Klondike	1	290	20	62
Super premium, avg	1	340	22	58
Dove Bar	1	350	22	57
Häagen-Dazs	1	390	27	62
Ice cream bombe	1	270	14	47
Ice cream cake (2 oz ice				
cream, 2 oz sauce):				
Butterscotch	1 slice	355	14	35
Chocolate	1 slice	385	15	38
Ice cream cake roll	1 slice	160	7	39
Ice cream cone:				
Chocolate	1 scoop	180	10	50
	2 scoops	360	20	50
Vanilla	1 scoop	170	8	42
	2 scoops	320	16	45
Cone Only				
Comet	1	40	0	0
Sugar	1	55	1	16

	AMOUNT	CALORIES	FAT-GRAMS	% FAT
Waffle				
Small	1	60	1	15
Large	1	200	3	14
Ice cream cup	1	15	0	0
Ice cream drumstick	1 sm	190	10	48
	1 lg	350	19	49
Ice cream pie (⅛ of 10" pie):				
Chocolate	1 slice	680	27	36
Pralines 'n' Cream	1 slice	810	46	51
Ice cream puff	1	225	7	28
Ice cream sandwich, avg:	1	170	6	32
Eskimo Pie, Original	1	140	10	64
Good Humor	1	160	5	28
Ice cream sundaes:				
Banana split (3 scoops ice cream w/ sauce, whipped cream, nuts, cherry)	1	1,350	76	51
Eskimo Boat	1	705	9	11
Two-scoop sundae:				
w/ butterscotch topping	1	535	25	42
w/ hot fudge	1	535	25	42
Chocolate ice cream, chocolate sauce, whipped cream, cherry	1	1,145	61	47

	AMOUNT	CALORIES	FAT-GRAMS	% FAT
Vanilla ice cream, chocolate sauce, whipped cream, cherry	1	1,085	61	50
Vanilla ice cream, strawberry syrup, whipped cream, nuts, cherry	1	1,065	57	48
Ice cream torte	4 oz	395	22	50
Ice milk (1% fat), avg:	½ cup	90	3	30
Carnation chocolate	½ cup	90	2	20
Borden Strawberry	½ cup	90	2	20
Weight Watchers Vanilla	½ cup	100	3	27
Ice milk, soft-serve, avg	½ cup	175	2	16
Ices:				
Italian ice	6 oz	140	0	0
Lemon ice	6 oz	140	0	0
Watermelon ice	6 oz	140	0	0
Mousse:				
Apricot	6 oz	360	3	7
Chocolate	1 cup	380	31	73
Peach chiffon	4 oz	200	5	22
Parisian cheese torte	1 slice	270	17	57
Pavlova	⅛ of 9" cake	220	11	45
Pie:				
Apple Betty	4 oz	215	5	21
Apple crisp (6" × 8")	4 oz	220	4	15
w/ cheese	1 serving	260	11	38

	AMOUNT	CALORIES	FAT-GRAMS	% FAT
Apple dumplings	1 apple	505	24	43
Apple streusel	4 oz	270	10	33
Apricot crunch				
(6" × 8")	1 serving	315	16	45
Black bottom pie	⅛ of			
	10" pie	380	16	38
Brown sugar pie	⅛ of			
	10" pie	585	25	38
Chiffon (⅛ of 10" pie)				
Banana	1 slice	555	37	60
Chocolate	1 slice	595	41	62
Egg nog	1 slice	655	40	55
Lime	1 slice	600	38	57
Mocha	1 slice	610	41	60
Orange	1 slice	605	38	57
Peach	1 slice	580	38	59
Peanut crunch	1 slice	700	42	54
Peppermint	1 slice	680	40	53
Pineapple	1 slice	580	38	59
Pumpkin	1 slice	665	38	51
Strawberry	1 slice	585	38	58
Chocolate pecan pie	1 slice	600	31	46
Chocolate silk pie	1 slice	600	40	60
Cobbler:				
Apple	5 oz	225	4	16
Blueberry	5 oz	250	4	14
Cherry	5 oz	260	4	14
Peach	5 oz	165	4	22
Pineapple-apricot	4 oz	220	4	16
Purple plum	5 oz	195	4	18

	AMOUNT	CALORIES	FAT-GRAMS	% FAT
Coconut custard pie	⅛ of 10" pie	365	18	45
Coconut macaroon pie	⅛ of 10" pie	635	36	51
Cranberry crunch (6" × 8")	1 serving	470	21	40
Cream cheese pie	1 slice	385	25	58
Cream pie (⅛ of 10" pie)	1 slice	435	30	62
Banana	1 slice	445	30	60
Bavarian	1 slice	315	17	49
Butterscotch	1 slice	400	20	45
Chocolate	1 slice	465	23	45
Coconut	1 slice	470	32	61
Date	1 slice	475	30	57
Raisin	1 slice	710	43	54
Crustless coconut pie	1 slice	380	18	42
Custard pie	1 slice	325	16	44
Date crunch (6" × 8")	1 serving	425	17	36
Fruit pie (⅛ of 10" pie)				
Apple	1 slice	495	20	36
Apricot	1 slice	455	20	40
Blackberry	1 slice	440	20	41
Blueberry	1 slice	435	20	41
Cherry	1 slice	465	20	39
Cherry glaze	1 slice	425	15	32
Peach	1 slice	480	20	37
Pineapple	1 slice	630	31	44
Strawberry	1 slice	440	20	41

	AMOUNT	CALORIES	FAT-GRAMS	% FAT
Strawberry parfait	1 slice	630	39	56
Strawberry rhubarb	1 slice	415	19	41
French silk pie. *See* Chocolate silk pie.				
Grasshopper pie	⅙ of 9" pie	575	35	55
Key lime pie	⅙ of 9" pie	460	19	37
Lemon chess pie	⅛ of 10" pie	600	23	35
Lemon meringue pie	⅛ of 10" pie	655	35	48
Lemon sponge chess pie	⅛ of 10" pie	655	35	47
Mincemeat pie	⅛ of 10" pie	510	20	35
Mud pie	⅛ of 10" pie	610	41	60
Peach crisp	4 oz	235	9	34
Peanut butter pie	⅛ of 10" pie	675	40	55
Pear crisp	4 oz	180	6	30
Pecan pie	⅛ of 10" pie	800	43	48
Pumpkin pie	⅛ of 10" pie	520	31	54
Raisin pie	⅛ of 10" pie	480	20	37

	AMOUNT	CALORIES	FAT-GRAMS	% FAT
Rhubarb crisp	½ cup	185	4	19
Shoofly pie	⅛ of 10" pie	705	38	49
Southern-style lemon icebox pie	⅛ of 10" pie	765	29	34
Pudding:				
Apple brown betty	½ cup	160	4	22
Banana meringue	½ cup	195	7	32
Blueberry crumb	1 sq	295	14	43
Bread	½ cup	175	5	26
Coconut	½ cup	185	7	34
Orange	½ cup	155	5	29
Brownie rice	½ cup	240	9	34
Butterscotch	½ cup	225	9	36
Caramel cake (4" × 6")	1 serving	315	11	31
Caramel raisin	½ cup	320	5	14
Chocolate	½ cup	185	6	29
Chocolate fudge	½ cup	370	10	24
Coconut	½ cup	235	8	31
Custard				
Baked	½ cup	155	7	41
Boiled	½ cup	165	7	38
Floating Island	½ cup	185	6	29
Fruit	½ cup	225	7	28
Baked	½ cup	360	18	45
Hunter	½ cup	325	16	44
Indian	½ cup	220	8	33
Lemon sponge	½ cup	220	10	41

	AMOUNT	CALORIES	FAT-GRAMS	% FAT
Marble cake	1 slice	160	11	61
Orange meringue	½ cup	210	3	13
Pear	½ cup	110	1	8
Pompadour	5 oz	280	9	29
Rice	½ cup	180	4	20
Baked	½ cup	240	7	26
Rice nut	½ cup	230	10	39
Tapioca	½ cup	150	4	24
Torte	½ cup	180	6	30
Vanilla	½ cup	265	8	27
Ricotta-strawberry manicotti w/ chocolate topping	1 shell	325	17	47
Shortcake:				
Peach shortcake	1 serving	425	20	42
Shortcake biscuit w/ fruit (3 oz biscuit, 2 oz fruit, 1 oz cream)	1 serving	270	17	57
Sorbet & ice cream, avg:	½ cup	190	8	38
Orange sorbet & vanilla ice cream	½ cup	190	8	38
Raspberry sorbet & vanilla ice cream	½ cup	180	7	35
Soufflé:				
Chocolate	4 oz	230	13	51
Coconut	4 oz	175	9	47
Orange	4 oz	155	8	46
Tiramisu	⅟₇ of 9" cake	255	17	60

	AMOUNT	CALORIES	FAT-GRAMS	% FAT
Vanilla cream square	1	90	5	50
White chocolate-hazelnut tartuffo	1	540	38	63
Yogurt, frozen, soft-serve, all flavors	½ cup	120	5	38
Low-fat, avg	½ cup	100	2	18
Nonfat, avg	½ cup	110	0	0
Zabaglione	4 oz	120	4	30

NONDAIRY DESSERTS

	AMOUNT	CALORIES	FAT-GRAMS	% FAT
Frozen fruit bar, avg:	1	80	0	0
Dole Cherry Bar	1	70	0	0
Minute Maid Grape Bar	1	60	0	0
Sunkist Orange Bar	1	70	0	0
Ice cream, avg	½ cup	150	8	48
Mocha mix Chocolate	½ cup	160	10	56
Strawberry	½ cup	140	7	45
Tofutti vanilla	½ cup	200	11	50
Light	½ cup	90	0	0
Soft-serve, vanilla	½ cup	160	8	45
Light	½ cup	90	1	10
Sherbert, avg	½ cup	110	1	8
Borden Lemon	½ cup	110	1	8
Borden Orange	½ cup	110	1	8
Sorbet, avg	½ cup	120	0	0
Dole Mandarin Orange	½ cup	110	0	0
Dole Peach	½ cup	120	0	0

	AMOUNT	CALORIES	FAT-GRAMS	% FAT
TOPPINGS				
Blueberries, fresh	2 tbsp	10	0	0
Blueberry sauce	2 tbsp	50	0	0
Butterfinger, crumbled	2 tbsp	130	5	35
Butterscotch topping	2 tbsp	140	1	6
Caramel topping	2 tbsp	140	1	6
Cherry topping	2 tbsp	100	0	0
Chocolate-chip cookie, crumbled	2 tbsp	130	6	42
Chocolate fudge topping	2 tbsp	125	5	36
Chocolate topping	2 tbsp	90	1	10
Coconut, shredded	2 tbsp	60	4	60
Fruit cocktail, juice-pack, canned	2 tbsp	15	0	0
Granola	2 tbsp	70	4	13
Hard sauce	2 tbsp	140	6	39
Heath bar, crumbled	2 tbsp	145	9	56
Hot fudge	2 tbsp	110	4	33
Lemon sauce	2 tbsp	60	2	30
M&M's				
Plain	2 tbsp	135	6	40
Peanut	2 tbsp	150	7	42
Maraschino cherry	1	10	0	0
Marshmallow	2 tbsp	120	0	0
Mixed nuts	2 tbsp	170	15	79
Nut topping	1 oz	180	16	80
Oreo cookies, crumbled	2 tbsp	140	6	39
Peanut butter caramel	2 tbsp	150	2	12

	AMOUNT	CALORIES	FAT-GRAMS	% FAT
Peanuts	2 tbsp	165	14	76
Pecans in syrup	2 tbsp	130	1	7
Pineapple topping	2 tbsp	100	0	0
Raisins	2 tbsp	55	0	0
Chocolate-covered	2 tbsp	120	5	38
Yogurt-covered	2 tbsp	135	6	40
Red raspberry topping	1 tbsp	50	0	0
Reese's Pieces	2 tbsp	140	6	39
Sprinkles, chocolate	1 tbsp	30	0	0
Strawberries, fresh	2 tbsp	5	0	0
Strawberry topping	2 tbsp	120	0	0
Walnuts in syrup	2 tbsp	130	1	7
Walnut topping	1 tbsp	90	5	50
Whipped toppings:				
Almond whipped cream	½ cup	175	17	88
Almond whipped topping	½ cup	90	5	49
Nondairy whipped topping	½ cup	95	8	76
Pressurized whipped cream	½ cup	75	7	84
Whipped cream, fresh	½ cup	205	22	96

EGGS & EGG DISHES

	AMOUNT	CALORIES	FAT-GRAMS	% FAT
Bacon & Egg Breakfast (3 strips bacon, 2 fried eggs, 1 cup hash brown potatoes, 2 slices toast w/ margarine)	I serving	900	54	54
Baked (shirred) eggs w/ cheese	2 eggs	265	22	74
Boiled egg	I	75	5	41
Breakfast pizza (eggs, olives, mushrooms, tomato)	⅙ of 12" pie	325	21	58
Calf brains & eggs	I serving	690	57	75
Canadian Bacon & Egg Breakfast (2 slices Canadian bacon, 2 fried eggs, 1 cup hash brown potatoes, 2 slices toast w/ margarine)	I serving	775	43	50
Cheesy egg roll-up tortilla	I	395	24	55
Chili relleno	I	340	24	64

	AMOUNT	CALORIES	FAT-GRAMS	% FAT
Curried eggs	5 oz	305	17	50
Deviled eggs	2 halves	145	13	80
Egg & bacon sandwich (w/ mayo)	1	503	32	57
Egg blintzes	2	186	6	29
Egg drop soup	6 oz	70	4	51
Egg foo yong (2-oz patties)	2 patties	210	15	65
Egg salad	½ cup	310	28	81
Egg salad pocket sandwich (w/ lettuce & tomato in pita)	1	255	8	28
Egg salad sandwich	1	255	9	32
Egg substitute, scrambled	2 eggs	130	6	43
Egg turnover w/ 2 oz cheese sauce	1 serving	470	34	65
Eggs à la goldenrod (eggs, toast, cream sauce)	5 oz	810	52	58
Eggs à la king	5 oz	690	43	56
Eggs à la Purgatory	2 eggs	220	14	57
Eggs w/ avocado sauce	2 eggs	400	33	74
Eggs Benedict (½ English muffin, 1 egg, ham, sauce)	1 serving	410	32	70
Eggs Benedict casserole	1 serving	395	28	64
Eggs w/ black beans & plantains	2 eggs	400	33	74
Eggs in cheese sauce	6 oz	355	22	56
Eggs on English muffin	2 eggs	280	17	55

	AMOUNT	CALORIES	FAT-GRAMS	% FAT
Eggs Florentine	2 tarts	530	40	68
Eggs Park Avenue (eggs, lox, sour cream, cream cheese, Hollandaise sauce)	6 oz	935	92	88
Eggs Romano (2 eggs, spinach, olives, Romano)	I serving	375	25	60
Eggs in shirts	3 eggs	440	40	82
Eggs Sojourn (2 eggs, crab & shrimp meat, English muffin, Hollandaise sauce)	I serving	1,790	159	80
Egg on tortilla (1 egg, 1 corn tortilla, cheese, salsa)	I serving	345	25	65
English muffin w/ egg, cheese & bacon	I serving	490	31	57
w/ egg, cheese & Canadian bacon	I serving	385	20	47
Fried egg	I	105	8	69
Fried Egg Breakfast (2 eggs) w/ 1 cup hash brown potatoes & 2 slices plain toast	I serving	560	29	47
w/ 1 cup hash brown potatoes, 3 oz ham & 2 slices plain toast	I serving	760	35	41

	AMOUNT	CALORIES	FAT-GRAMS	% FAT
w/ 1 cup hash brown potatoes & 2 slices toast w/ margarine	I serving	690	39	51
w/ 1 cup hash brown potatoes 3 strips bacon, 2 slices toast w/ margarine	I serving	795	47	53
w/ 2 pancakes w/ syrup & margarine, 2 sausage links & 2 strips bacon	I serving	1,050	52	43
w/ 1 cup hash brown potatoes, 4 sausage links & 2 slices toast w/ margarine	I serving	1,040	70	61
w/ 3 pancakes w/ syrup & margarine, 3 sausage links & 3 strips bacon	I serving	1,490	76	46
Frittata w/ mushrooms	3 eggs	310	23	67
w/ zucchini, cheese & artichokes	3 eggs	585	47	72
Ham & Egg Breakfast (2 fried eggs, 1 cup hash brown potatoes, 3 oz ham & 2 slices toast w/ margarine)	I serving	760	35	41
w/ 3 pancakes w/ syrup & margarine	I serving	1,530	57	34

	AMOUNT	CALORIES	FAT-GRAMS	% FAT
Ham & egg salad sandwich	1	305	15	44
Huevos con queso in tortilla (2 eggs, cheese, tortilla sauce)	1 serving	745	53	64
Huevos leone (bacon omelet w/ tortilla)	10 oz	565	42	67
Huevos rancheros	6 oz	390	25	58
Hungarian gulyas (egg, yogurt, ham, cheese, sunflower seeds)	5 oz	425	34	72
Oeufs Antoine (eggs, bacon, capers, English muffin, Mornay sauce)	6 oz	705	50	64
Omelets (3 eggs):				
Bacon omelet	1	375	28	67
Basque omelet (w/ peppers, onion, tomato)	1	430	36	75
Cheese omelet	1	355	26	66
Cheese Omelet Breakfast (1 cup hash brown potatoes, 3 strips bacon, 2 slices toast w/ margarine)	1 serving	940	57	55
w/ 3 pancakes w/ syrup & margarine	1 serving	1,710	79	42

	AMOUNT	CALORIES	FAT-GRAMS	% FAT
Farmer-style omelet (eggs, onion, ham, potatoes)	1	405	30	67
Ham omelet	1	295	21	64
Mushroom omelet	1	300	22	66
Plain omelet	1	330	21	57
Spanish omelet (w/ Creole sauce)	1	350	25	64
Western omelet (eggs, bacon, ham, onion, peppers)	1	355	25	63
Poached egg:	1	75	5	41
Creamy poached egg (1 egg on ½ English muffin w/ cheese sauce)	1 serving	325	20	56
Poached eggs Henri (eggs, toast, Canadian bacon, asparagus, Hollandaise sauce)	6 oz	690	55	72
Sausage & Egg Breakfast (2 fried eggs, 4 links sausage, 1 cup hash brown potatoes, 2 slices toast w/ margarine)	1 serving	1,030	71	62
w/ 3 pancakes w/ syrup & margarine	1 serving	1,750	83	43

EGGS/EGG DISHES

	AMOUNT	CALORIES	FAT-GRAMS	% FAT
Scrambled eggs				
(2 large eggs)	l serving	200	15	68
w/ 2 oz ham	l serving	275	21	68
w/ herbs	l serving	205	15	66
w/ mushrooms	l serving	210	15	64
w/ smoked salmon	l serving	305	19	56
Scrambled Egg Breakfast				
(2 large eggs)				
w/ 1 cup hash brown potatoes & 2 slices plain toast	l serving	640	26	37
w/ 1 cup hash brown potatoes, 2 oz ham & 2 slices plain toast	l serving	740	29	35
w/ 1 cup hash brown potatoes & 2 slices toast w/ margarine	l serving	770	36	42
w/ 1 cup hash brown potatoes, 3 strips bacon & 2 slices toast w/ margarine	l serving	875	44	45
w/ 2 pancakes w/ syrup & margarine, 2 sausage links & 2 strips bacon	l serving	1,130	49	39
w/ 1 cup hash brown potatoes, 4 sausage links & 2 slices toast w/ margarine	l serving	1,120	67	54

	AMOUNT	CALORIES	FAT GRAMS	% FAT
w/ 3 pancakes w/ syrup & margarine, 3 sausage links & 3 strips bacon	1 serving	1,570	73	42
Scrambled egg substitute (= 2 eggs)	1 serving	130	6	43
w/ 1 cup hash brown potatoes & 2 slices plain toast	1 serving	480	18	35
w/ 1 cup hash brown potatoes, 2 oz ham & 2 slices plain toast	1 serving	580	22	34
Soufflé:				
Cheese	6 oz	325	24	66
Spinach	6 oz	320	18	51
Stracciatella (egg & cheese soup)	8 oz	65	3	42
Swiss eggs (3 eggs, Swiss cheese, Gruyère)	3 eggs	505	44	78
Zucchini & egg crepes	2 crepes	445	29	58

GARNISHES & ENTRÉE ACCOMPANIMENTS

	AMOUNT	CALORIES	FAT-GRAMS	% FAT
Apples:				
Apple fritter rings	3 fritters	340	14	37
Caramel apples	4 oz	150	4	24
Cinnamon apple ring	1 serving	50	1	21
Escalloped apples	4 oz	180	6	30
French apple puffs	2	260	15	52
Glazed apples	2 slices	175	6	31
Bananas, fried	2 halves	205	12	53
Blueberry sinkers	2	260	14	48
Fritters:				
Apple fritter rings	3 fritters	340	14	37
Cherry fritters	2	260	15	52
Royal Hawaiian fritters	2	265	15	51
Glazed peach	½ peach	130	2	14
Spiced fruit	1 serving	110	0	0
Yorkshire pudding (3" square)	1 serving	171	10	52

MEATS & MEAT DISHES

	AMOUNT	CALORIES	FAT-GRAMS	% FAT
BEEF				
Beef & green bean casserole	8 oz	245	14	51
Beef, biscuit & gravy	1 serving	480	31	58
Beef bologna sandwich w/o mayo	1	305	16	47
Beef Burgundy	6 oz	300	10	30
Beef casserole w/ vegetables, rice & sauce	2 cups	550	24	39
Beef Creole	6 oz	285	9	28
Beef curry	6 oz	275	9	29
Beef goulash	6 oz	300	11	33
Beef jerky	1 oz	110	4	33
Beef kabob teriyaki	1 kabob	380	14	33
Beef noodle casserole	8 oz	420	19	40
Beef paprikash	6 oz	340	15	40
Beef pot pie	8 oz	840	62	66
Beef roulade w/ 2 oz sauce	1 serving	460	24	47
Beef stew	2 cups	440	20	43
Beef Stroganoff	2 cups	690	50	65
Beef turnover	1	565	42	67

	AMOUNT	CALORIES	FAT-GRAMS	% FAT
Beef Wellington	8 oz	650	36	50
Beef w/ oyster sauce	6 oz	270	16	54
Brains, pan-fried:				
Beef	3.5 oz	200	15	68
Calf	3.5 oz	125	9	65
Braised beef w/ gravy (6 oz meat, 2.5 oz gravy)	1 serving	565	28	44
Brisket of beef	4 oz	480	25	47
Cannelloni w/ ground beef & cheese	1 pc	420	30	64
Cheeseburger (w/o mayo or mayo-type dressing)	1	320	15	42
Double	1	545	28	46
Extra-large	1	610	33	49
Chicken-fried steak	4 oz	580	41	64
Chili:				
Chili con carne	8 oz	255	8	28
Chili Santa Fe	10 oz	340	17	45
Chili verde	8 oz	270	15	50
Chili w/ macaroni	8 oz	255	6	21
Chipped beef:	1 oz	45	1	20
Chipped beef w/ egg	6 oz	235	15	57
Chipped beef w/ macaroni	8 oz	315	17	48
Creamed chipped beef	6 oz	300	20	60
Corned beef	3.5 oz	250	19	68
Corned beef hash	1 cup	375	24	58

	AMOUNT	CALORIES	FAT-GRAMS	% FAT
Corned beef on rye				
sandwich	1	370	19	46
Deli-size (8 oz)	1	800	60	68
Flank steak, broiled				
Lean & fat	8 oz	580	36	56
Lean only	8 oz	560	34	54
Green pepper stuffed				
w/ beef & rice	1 med	260	14	48
Golabki (cabbage roll)	1	260	13	45
Hamburger (w/o mayo or				
mayo-type dressing	1	275	12	39
Double	1	460	22	43
Extra-large	1	510	27	48
Hamburger pie	8 oz	475	28	53
Hash:				
Beef	8 oz	390	23	53
Corned beef	8 oz	320	17	48
Red flannel	8 oz	425	22	46
Hot dog, regular	1	240	15	54
w/ chili	1	325	18	49
Lasagna	1 pc	400	20	45
Liver, sautéed	8 oz	720	46	57
Macaroni, beef &				
tomato casserole	8 oz	285	13	41
Meatballs:				
Italian meatball	1 med	75	5	60
Meatballs in				
sour cream gravy				
(1" meatballs,				
1.5 oz gravy)	3 meatballs	370	23	56

	AMOUNT	CALORIES	FAT-GRAMS	% FAT
Meatballs Stroganoff (1" meatballs, 2 oz sauce)	3 meatballs	370	23	56
Porcupine meatballs (1" each)	3	275	14	46
Swedish meatballs (1" meatballs, 1 oz sauce)	3 meatballs	285	16	50
Meat loaf	4 oz	295	17	52
Mexican-style beef:				
Burrito	1	390	14	32
w/ sour cream		440	20	41
Carne Asada	6 oz	365	25	61
Carnitas de Res (sirloin strips, vegetables, sauce)	6 oz	305	16	47
Chimichanga (beef, cheese, tortilla, sour cream)	1	660	44	60
Enchilada w/ sour cream	1	435	30	62
Fajita (beef, peppers, onion, tortilla)	1	510	30	53
w/ 2 tbsp guacamole & 2 tbsp sour cream		615	40	59
Flauta (6" tortilla, beef filling)	1	255	15	53
w/ 2 tbsp guacamole & 2 tbsp sour cream	1	355	25	63
Quesadilla (6")	1	430	26	54

	AMOUNT	CALORIES	FAT-GRAMS	% FAT
Short ribs w/ chipotle sauce	1 meaty rib	580	25	39
Sopito	1	490	29	53
Taco (1 corn tortilla, ½ cup filling)	1	280	16	51
w/ 2 tbsp guacamole & 2 tbsp sour cream	385	26	61	
Tamale pie	8 oz	310	13	38
Tamales (2 small w/ sauce)	1 serving	345	20	52
Tostada (beef, beans, cheese, olives, avocado, sour cream) (8")	1	1,005	64	57
Oriental-style beef:				
Bahmi Goreng w/ sauce (beef, noodles, vegetables)	main dish	465	16	31
per 1 tbsp peanut sauce	add	40	3	68
Cashew beef	main dish	670	44	59
Chinese beef & green pepper stir-fry	6 oz	295	11	34
Ginger beef stir-fry	6 oz	305	10	29
Mongolian beef (w/ green onions, rice noodles)	main dish	480	22	41
Noodles & beef w/ black bean sauce	main dish	680	36	48
Oyster sauce beef	6 oz	270	16	54

	AMOUNT	CALORIES	FAT-GRAMS	% FAT
Peking beef	main dish	435	29	60
Stir-fried beef (w/ onions, peppers, snow peas, mushrooms)	7 oz	345	22	57
w/ bok choy	main dish	405	26	57
w/ broccoli	7 oz	320	19	54
w/ napa cabbage	main dish	385	23	54
w/ oyster sauce over noodles	8 oz	435	20	41
w/ snow peas & water chestnuts	8 oz	435	29	60
Szechuan beef	7 oz	350	17	44
Pastrami sandwich	1	660	53	72
Philly beef sandwich (roast beef, onions, mushrooms, melted cheese & dressing on French roll)	1	820	33	36
Ragout of beef	main dish	640	29	40
Reuben sandwich	1	530	33	56
Deli-size (8 oz)	1	1,300	75	52
Roasts:				
Pot roast (2.5 oz beef, 2 oz gravy)	1 serving	245	12	44
Prime rib roast (lean only)	8 oz	405	23	51
Prime rib roast, blackened	8 oz	585	44	68
Roast boneless rib of beef	8 oz	405	23	50

	AMOUNT	CALORIES	FAT-GRAMS	% FAT
Roast tenderloin of beef	3 oz	155	7	40
Standing rib roast	8 oz	405	23	51
Roast beef sandwich				
w/o mayo	1	345	14	36
w/ cheese	1	400	18	40
Sauerbraten (4 oz meat, 4 oz gravy)	1 serving	590	36	55
Short ribs				
Barbecued	1 rib	560	48	85
Braised	1 rib	590	51	77
Sloppy joe	5 oz	200	12	54
Spaghetti & meat sauce	1 cup	320	17	48
Steaks:				
Bavarian beef steak	4 oz	285	16	51
Beef steak teriyaki	4 oz	310	15	44
Beef tips & eggplant				
w/ tomato sauce	4 oz	400	16	36
Braised beef steak	4 oz	230	11	43
w/ onions	4 oz	275	13	43
Braised cubed beef	6 oz	275	9	30
Chopped sirloin steak	5 oz	225	9	36
Delmonico steak (choice)				
Lean & fat	8 oz	570	44	70
Lean only	8 oz	370	20	49
Filet mignon (prime)				
Lean & fat	8 oz	450	37	74
Lean only	8 oz	385	20	47
London broil	5 oz	300	22	66

	AMOUNT	CALORIES	FAT-GRAMS	% FAT
New York steak, lean only	8 oz	385	20	47
New York steak sandwich (grilled lean New York steak on French roll)	1	340	13	34
Pepper steak	5 oz	245	15	55
Porterhouse steak (choice)				
Lean & fat	8 oz	650	52	72
Lean only	8 oz	360	18	45
Rib-eye steak (choice)				
Lean & fat	8 oz	570	44	70
Lean only	8 oz	370	20	49
Round steak Italienne	4 oz	210	9	38
Salisbury steak	5 oz	335	20	53
w/ tomato sauce		355	22	56
Sirloin steak (prime)				
Lean & fat	8 oz	655	27	37
Lean only	8 oz	310	12	35
w/ béarnaise sauce, mushrooms & truffles	6 oz	805	61	68
w/ escargots (broiled beef loin steak, escargot)	1	675	41	55
Steak sandwich (3 oz)	1	325	12	33
Skirt steak (lean only)	6 oz	385	22	51

	AMOUNT	CALORIES	FAT-GRAMS	% FAT
Spanish-style steak				
(w/ Creole sauce)	4 oz	245	11	40
Steak au poivre	10 oz	670	38	51
Steak Barrington				
(bacon-wrapped,				
broiled ground				
round)	8 oz	510	35	62
Steak fajita wrap	1	510	25	44
Steak Oscar	6 oz	805	61	68
Steak teriyaki	4 oz	325	15	41
Stuffed flank steak	5 oz	330	19	52
Swiss steak	4 oz	205	13	47
w/ gravy	4 oz	300	18	54
w/ sour cream	5 oz	260	22	77
T-bone steak (choice)				
Lean & fat	8 oz	735	55	68
Lean only	8 oz	485	23	43
Tenderloin (prime)				
Lean & fat	5.5 oz	450	37	74
Lean only	8 oz	385	20	47
Tenderloin tips				
(on toast points,				
w/ mushrooms &				
Burgundy sauce)	5 oz	485	28	52
Top loin steak (prime)				
Lean & fat	10 oz	805	63	71
Lean only	8 oz	425	24	51
Tournedos à la crème				
(beef tournedo,				
cream sauce)	8 oz	635	43	61

	AMOUNT	CALORIES	FAT-GRAMS	% FAT
Tournedos Messina (beef fillet, bread, chicken liver pâté, artichokes, mushrooms)	8 oz	730	49	60
Stews:				
Beef stew	8 oz	315	12	35
Beef stew Bordelaise	8 oz	375	17	40
Irish stew	8 oz	280	7	22
Old-fashioned beef stew w/ dumplings	8 oz	745	30	36
Stuffed cabbage	1	330	20	54
Stuffed pepper	½ pepper	320	20	56
w/ cheese		525	30	51
Tomato beef	main dish	310	18	52
Tongue, smoked	2.5 oz	260	19	65
GAME				
Buffalo, roasted	4 oz	140	2	15
Stewed rabbit	¼ rabbit	380	16	38
Venison chop, marinated	1	315	12	34
Venison pot roast	4 oz	330	12	33
Venison sauerbraten	4 oz	235	9	34
LAMB				
BBQ lamb ribs	1	265	11	37
Boiled lamb w/ dill sauce	6 oz	300	15	45
Braised lamb shank	1	515	33	58

	AMOUNT	CALORIES	FAT-GRAMS	% FAT
Braised lamb shoulder chop	1	275	14	46
Carbonnade of lamb	6 oz	290	13	40
Chili:				
Chili Santa Fe	8 oz	345	17	44
New Mexican green chili	8 oz	340	16	43
Chopped lamb, lean & fat, cooked	4 oz	195	13	60
Crown roast of lamb w/ stuffing	2 chops	745	34	91
Greek-style lamb w/ orzo (4 oz meat, 2 oz orzo)	1 serving	415	12	26
Ground lamb, lean & fat, cooked	4 oz	155	10	58
Hunter-style lamb (w/ garlic, rosemary)	7 oz	495	41	75
Lamb & artichoke w/ avgolemono sauce (1 lamb shank, 3 oz vegetable, sauce)	1 serving	310	11	32
Lamb & couscous	6 oz	345	14	36
Lamb chop w/ bone, lean & fat, broiled	1 medium	255	21	74
Lamb curry	6 oz	325	18	50
Lamb fricassee	6 oz	265	10	34
Lamb patty	4 oz	235	15	57
Lamb pilaf	6 oz	375	13	31
Lamb pot pie	8 oz	370	19	46

MEATS/MEAT DISHES

	AMOUNT	CALORIES	FAT-GRAMS	% FAT
Lamb riblets	2	390	18	41
Lamb Salonika (w/ mushrooms & cream sauce)	6 oz	280	18	58
Lamb scallops				
à la crème (lamb leg, mushrooms, onions, cream sauce)	6 oz	260	16	56
Provençal (lamb leg, onion, garlic, wine tomatoes)	6 oz	285	12	38
Lamb stew	6 oz	310	21	61
Leg of lamb:				
Leg of lamb roast	3 oz	180	7	35
w/ potatoes & vegetables	6 oz	455	16	32
Stuffed leg of lamb, en croute	6 oz	665	36	49
Moussaka	8 oz	685	33	43
Navarin of spring lamb	6 oz	485	28	52
New Mexican green chili	8 oz	340	16	43
Rack of lamb	4 oz	470	34	65
Roast lamb shoulder	6 oz	250	16	57
Stuffed	6 oz	680	34	45
Rolled braised lamb shoulder	6 oz	645	36	50
Russian bitki lamb patties	4 oz	515	36	63
Shepherd's pie	10 oz	330	12	33
Shish kabob	1 kabob	305	16	48

	AMOUNT	CALORIES	FAT-GRAMS	% FAT
Stuffed breast of lamb	6 oz	335	13	35
Stuffed Turks (½ stuffed green pepper)	1 serving	255	13	46

PORK

	AMOUNT	CALORIES	FAT-GRAMS	% FAT
Bacon				
Medium slice	2 strips	70	5	71
Thick slice	2 strips	100	8	72
Bacon, Canadian	2 slices	85	4	42
Bacon & Egg Breakfast (3 strips bacon, 2 fried eggs, 1 cup hash brown potatoes, 2 slices toast w/ margarine)	1 serving	900	54	54
Bacon, lettuce & tomato sandwich (3 slices bacon) w/ mayo	1	420	21	45
Bratwurst, cooked	1	255	22	78
Canadian Bacon & Egg Breakfast (2 slices Canadian bacon, 2 fried eggs, 1 cup hash brown potatoes, 2 slices toast w/ margarine)	1 serving	775	43	50
Cashew pork & pea pods	main dish	555	21	34
Chitterlings, cooked	1 oz	200	21	95
Corn dog	1	330	20	55

	AMOUNT	CALORIES	FAT-GRAMS	% FAT
Fish-flavored pork	main dish	435	24	50
Ham:				
Baked ham	2.5 oz	155	8	46
Creamed ham	6 oz	285	18	56
Croquettes	1	220	14	57
Escalloped ham & cabbage (w/ creamy cheese sauce)	8 oz	390	23	53
Escalloped ham & macaroni (w/ cheese sauce)	8 oz	420	21	45
Ham à la king (w/ mushrooms, cream sauce)	6 oz	270	16	53
Ham & cheese melt on hamburger bun	1	320	17	48
Ham & cheese sandwich	1	390	24	55
Ham & lima beans	8 oz	280	6	19
Ham & noodles au gratin	8 oz	465	27	52
Ham & potatoes au gratin	8 oz	400	22	49
Ham & sweet potatoes w/ apples	8 oz	345	7	18
Ham crepes w/ 2 oz sauce	2 crepes	400	16	36
Ham, macaroni & tomato casserole	8 oz	255	9	10

	AMOUNT	CALORIES	FAT-GRAMS	% FAT
Ham patty	5 oz raw	305	14	41
Ham roll au gratin (ham, broccoli, toast, sauce)	main dish	670	39	52
Ham salad sandwich	1	320	17	48
Ham sandwich				
w/ mayo	1	365	19	47
w/o mayo	1	285	16	51
Ham shortcake (ham, corn bread, sauce)	8 oz	355	15	38
Ham steak, grilled	3 oz	180	9	45
Honey glazed ham steak, baked	3 oz	240	10	37
Roast fresh ham	2.5 oz	105	5	42
Hungarian pork goulash	8 oz	295	19	58
Hot dog	1	340	18	48
Hot pork sandwich w/ gravy	1	420	18	38
Hot roast beef sandwich w/ gravy	1	420	15	32
Italian sausage sandwich (w/ peppers, onion & olive on Italian roll)	1	620	44	64
Liverwurst sandwich	1	550	34	56
Moo goo gai pan	main dish	545	15	25
Moo shu pork	main dish	630	38	54
Mexicali pork chili	8 oz	590	41	63
Noodles w/ pork & peanut sauce	main dish	580	25	39

	AMOUNT	CALORIES	FAT-GRAMS	% FAT
Polsa (Swedish hash)	10 oz	200	7	32
Pork & Spanish rice	8 oz	335	13	35
Pork burrito	1	385	24	56
w/ sour cream		435	30	62
Pork chimichanga (pork, cheese tortilla, sour cream)	1	665	44	60
Pork chops				
BBQ	1 chop	390	25	57
Beer-braised, w/ brown sauce	1 chop	655	45	62
Creole-style	1 chop	310	13	38
in orange sauce	1 chop	335	25	67
Italian-style, w/ fried potatoes	1 serving	595	28	43
Smoked	1 chop	290	11	34
Stuffed (bread dressing)	1 chop	490	36	66
w/ Madeira sauce	1 chop	505	31	55
Pork chop suey	8 oz	195	10	46
Pork chow mein	6 oz	270	18	59
Pork cutlet, breaded	1	260	10	35
Pork fried rice	1 cup	355	17	43
Pork kabob	1	345	12	31
Pork loaf	4 oz	285	13	41
Pork loin w/ gravy	4 oz	160	9	51
Pork meatballs w/ ginger glaze	6 sm	235	9	35
Pork, noodle & cheese casserole	8 oz	390	20	46

	AMOUNT	CALORIES	FAT-GRAMS	% FAT
Pork ragout	8 oz	600	25	37
Pork, shrimp, vegetables				
& rice (Thai-style)	main dish	565	30	48
Pork stew	8 oz	600	25	37
Pork taco (1 corn tortilla,				
⅓ cup filling)	1	280	16	51
w/ 2 tbsp sour cream		335	22	59
w/ 2 tbsp sour cream				
& 2 tbsp guacamole		385	26	61
Pork tenderloin				
in mushroom				
cream sauce	4 oz	260	14	48
Oriental	6 oz	285	16	57
w/ apple-celery				
dressing	main dish	345	18	47
w/ peppers & onions	4 oz	280	13	42
Pork tetrazzini	1 cup	345	20	52
Roast loin of pork,				
bone in	4 oz	275	16	52
Roast suckling pig	6 oz	410	21	46
Salami sandwich	1	480	34	64
Sausages:				
Bockwurst	4 oz	260	24	83
Bratwurst	4 oz	340	28	74
Chorizo				
(Mexican sausage)	4 oz	300	24	71
Italian sausage	4 oz	265	24	82
w/ green peppers		295	24	76
Italian sausage,				
braised w/ polenta	1 sausage	505	30	53

	AMOUNT	CALORIES	FAT-GRAMS	% FAT
Knockwurst				
(pork & beef)	3.5 oz	280	15	48
Polish sausage, fresh	4 oz	230	20	78
Sausage links				
(1 oz each)	1	110	11	90
Sausage patty	3 oz	330	33	90
Scallopini à la Marsala	1 cutlet	300	18	54
Scrapple (2 slices)	3 oz	255	8	28
Spareribs:				
BBQ spareribs	8 oz	645	43	60
Hawaiian spareribs	8 oz	600	43	64
Spareribs & sauerkraut				
(8 oz ribs,				
4 oz sauerkraut)	1 serving	595	43	65
Stir-fried pork				
w/ vegetables	main dish	435	24	50
Swedish meatballs				
(1" each)	6	585	37	57
Sweet & sour pork	8 oz	255	8	28
Sweet & sour pork				
balls (1" each)	3	225	7	28
Szechuan pork	main dish	300	20	60
Twice-cooked pork	main dish	300	20	60

VEAL

	AMOUNT	CALORIES	FAT-GRAMS	% FAT
Braised veal shank				
w/ risotto	1 shank	495	11	20
Braised veal w/ prosciutto				
& escarole	7 oz	360	18	45
Breaded veal cutlet	4 oz	385	15	35

	AMOUNT	CALORIES	FAT-GRAMS	% FAT
Calf's liver	6 oz	445	33	68
Hungarian veal paprikash (veal, onions, cream sauce)	6 oz	370	24	58
Medallion of veal sauté (veal loin, mushrooms, cream sauce)	4 oz	535	35	59
Osso buco (braised veal)	1 shank	875	39	40
Roast veal	3 oz	145	5	31
Saltimbocca	2 rolls	415	21	45
Stir-fried veal w/ peppers	8 oz	385	29	68
Swiss-style shredded veal (w/ mushrooms, shallots, cream sauce)	6 oz	415	26	32
Veal chop in sour cream	1 chop	345	19	50
Veal Cordon Bleu (veal, ham, Swiss cheese)	4 oz	440	27	55
Veal curry	6 oz	390	26	60
Veal cutlet:	4 oz	285	12	38
Breaded	4 oz	385	15	35
Italienne (cutlet, peppers, tomato sauce)	4 oz	325	14	39
Marsala (cutlet, prosciutto, mushrooms, wine sauce)	1 cutlet	455	31	62

	AMOUNT	CALORIES	FAT-GRAMS	% FAT
Messina-style (sautéed veal, bread, ham, tomato sauce)	1 cutlet	530	28	48
Swiss-style (sautéed veal, tomatoes, mushrooms)	1 cutlet	360	11	28
Veal fricassee	8 oz	450	21	42
Veal goulash	6 oz	305	15	44
Veal kidneys in red wine	5 oz	265	19	64
Veal loaf	1 slice	270	17	57
Veal Marengo (veal, pasta, mushrooms, tomato sauce)	6 oz	340	12	31
Veal Marsala	4 oz	285	20	63
Veal meatballs (w/ tomato sauce & ½ cup rice)	8 oz	430	22	46
Veal Oscar (w/ crab, asparagus, Hollandaise sauce)	4 oz	910	73	72
Veal Parmigiana (cutlet, mozzarella, tomato sauce, Parmesan)	6 oz	590	30	46
Veal piccata	4 oz	265	12	41
Veal Piemontese (sautéed veal, artichokes, cream sauce)	6 oz	480	39	73

	AMOUNT	CALORIES	FAT-GRAMS	% FAT
Veal Provençal (sautéed veal, cream, Madeira sauce)	1 cutlet	280	16	51
Veal roll (w/ bacon & sour cream)	1 roll	460	36	71
Veal scallopini	8 oz	590	29	44
Veal scallops & rice casserole (w/ onions, celery, carrots & peas)	8 oz	285	10	32
Veal schnitzel (4 oz patties)	2 patties	425	30	64
Veal steak w/ eggplant (mozzarella & tomato sauce)	4 oz	755	63	75
Veal stew	8 oz	240	7	26
Veal sweetbread	2 pcs	765	25	29
Wiener schnitzel	4 oz	425	30	64

PASTA & PASTA DISHES

The pasta dishes in this section are based on cooked yields. A 5-ounce portion of cooked pasta measures approximately 1 cup; a 4-ounce portion of sauce measures approximately ½ cup. The combination of 5 ounces of pasta and 4 ounces of sauce, yielding a 9-ounce portion, is a modest serving. In many restaurants, the portion served might be one and a half to two times that size.

	AMOUNT	CALORIES	FAT-GRAMS	% FAT
Cannelloni w/ ground beef & cheese	1 piece	420	30	64
Average serving	10 oz	625	37	53
Kuchen, cheese	8 oz	440	21	43
Kugel w/ raisins	4 oz	395	12	27
Lasagna:				
Seafood lasagna (pasta, halibut, salmon, shrimp, vegetables, tomato sauce, cheese)	10 oz	620	38	55
Traditional lasagna (pasta, meat sauce, ricotta, mozzarella)	10 oz	625	37	53

	AMOUNT	CALORIES	FAT-GRAMS	% FAT
Macaroni:				
Calico macaroni (pasta, tomato, bacon, peas, cheese) (4" × 6")	1 serving	270	9	30
Cheese & tomato casserole	6 oz	240	11	41
Macaroni & cheese	¾ cup	315	19	54
Macaroni-stuffed green pepper w/ cheese	1	335	19	51
Macaroni-stuffed tomato w/ cheese	1	340	19	50
Manicotti (pasta, ricotta, Parmesan, spinach, tomato sauce, mozzarella)	10 oz	720	24	30
Mostaccioli w/ gorgonzola & tomatoes	10 oz	540	19	32
Noodles:				
Buttered noodles	3 oz	135	3	20
Noodles Alfredo (w/ cream sauce)	9 oz	1,000	61	55
Noodles Lyonnaise (w/ butter & Parmesan)	3 oz	130	4	27
Noodles Mizar (w/ cottage cheese & sour cream)	3 oz	165	8	43
Noodles Romanoff (w/ sour cream, butter & Parmesan)	1 cup	325	22	61

	AMOUNT	CALORIES	FAT-GRAMS	% FAT
Noodle, salmon & mushroom casserole	12oz	595	32	48
Poppy seed noodles (w/ butter & slivered almonds)	3 oz	160	6	34
Tuna noodle casserole	8 oz	300	12	36
Noodles, Oriental-style:				
Bahmi Goreng (meat, Chinese noodles, vegetables)	main dish	465	16	31
w/ peanut sauce	*add per 1 tbsp*	40	3	68
Bean threads, braised w/ pork & vegetables (Ants on a Tree)	main dish	395	21	48
Chop suey				
w/ chicken	8 oz	255	10	35
w/ pork	8 oz	195	10	46
Chow mein				
Beef	1 cup	300	17	51
Chicken	1 cup	255	10	35
Pork	6 oz	270	18	60
Seafood, meat & vegetable				
Pan-fried	main dish	680	36	48
w/ soft noodles	12 oz	565	30	48
Shrimp	1 cup	220	10	41
Chow mein noodles	½ cup	230	5	20
Oriental noodles, no fat added	1 cup	95	1	9

	AMOUNT	CALORIES	FAT-GRAMS	% FAT
Oriental noodles w/ chicken, shiitake mushrooms & sauce	10 oz	425	31	66
Oriental noodles w/ pork & peanut sauce	main dish	580	25	39
Pasta w/ chicken & vegetables in Szechuan sauce	12 oz	615	22	32
Rice noodles w/ pork, shrimp & vegetables	main dish	565	30	48
Szechuan noodles w/ Chinese cabbage & snow peas	8 oz	305	16	47
Szechuan noodles w/ Chinese cabbage, snow peas & scallops	10 oz	405	30	66
Thai noodles w/ pork, shrimp & chicken	main dish	555	15	24
Pansotti w/ butter sauce	10 oz	605	30	45
Pasta:				
Plain (5 oz)	1 cup	210	1	4
w/ anchovies, garlic & olive oil	9 oz	705	30	38
w/ beans	1 cup	300	8	24
w/ chicken & mushrooms in cream sauce	12 oz	1,145	64	50
w/ chicken & pancetta in spicy red sauce topped w/ mozzarella	14 oz	975	55	51

	AMOUNT	CALORIES	FAT-GRAMS	% FAT
w/ cream sauce & prosciutto	12 oz	1,040	61	53
w/ cream sauce & seafood (mussels, scallops, clams, crab)	12 oz	1,260	63	45
w/ cream sauce, salmon & sun-dried tomatoes	12 oz	1,200	79	59
w/ eggplant, tomatoes, garlic, cheese & olive oil	12 oz	705	30	38
w/ fresh tomatoes, basil & garlic	12 oz	520	11	19
w/ fresh tomatoes, basil, garlic & olive oil	12 oz	760	29	34
w/ ham, peas, Parmesan & butter	12 oz	555	21	34
w/ Italian sausage, spaghetti sauce & Sicilian peppers	14 oz	795	39	45
w/ marinara sauce	10 oz	295	5	15
w/ marinara & mushroom sauce	10 oz	330	7	19
w/ meatballs & tomato sauce (5 oz pasta, 5 oz sauce, 2 small meatballs)	13 oz	630	20	29
w/ meat sauce (5 oz pasta, 5 oz sauce)	10 oz	410	11	24

	AMOUNT	CALORIES	FAT-GRAMS	% FAT
w/ meat sauce, mozzarella & Parmesan	8 oz	405	22	49
w/ mushrooms & light cream sauce	1 cup	280	13	42
w/ pesto & seafood (clams, mussels, scallops, crab)	12 oz	1,010	45	42
w/ prawns in garlic, wine & plum tomatoes	14 oz	915	42	41
w/ red clam sauce	12 oz	485	9	17
w/ spicy red sauce & seafood (mussels, clams, scallops, crab)	12 oz	545	14	23
w/ sweet peppers, basil, tomato & olive oil	¾ cup	170	8	42
w/ tomato sauce, meatless	10 oz	320	6	17
w/ tomatoes in spicy sauce (crushed red peppers) & Romano	¾ cup	290	9	25
w/ tomatoes in spicy sauce w/ pancetta	10 oz	655	39	54
w/ tuna, anchovies, olives, tomatoes, olive oil & mozzarella	12 oz	695	26	34
w/ veal in cream sauce	14 oz	665	25	34
w/ white clam sauce	14 oz	985	47	43

	AMOUNT	CALORIES	FAT-GRAMS	% FAT
Pasta all'Amatriciana (pasta, bacon, olive oil, white wine, tomatoes, Romano)	10 oz	655	39	53
Pasta alla Carbonara	9 oz	675	34	45
Pasta alla Francese (pasta, ham, peas, Parmesan, butter)	10 oz	555	21	34
Pasta alla Puttanesca (pasta, tomato sauce, olives, capers, garlic, basil)	8 oz	440	15	30
Pasta alla Romana (pasta, bacon, butter, Romano)	9 oz	675	34	45
Pasta Bolognese (5 oz pasta, 5 oz sauce)	10 oz	410	14	31
Pasta Capperei (pasta, basil, tomato sauce, olives, capers, garlic)	8 oz	440	15	30
Pasta e fagioli (pasta & beans)	1 cup	300	8	24
Pasta Florentine (pasta, spinach, pine nuts, anchovies, béchamel sauce)	14 oz	685	23	30
Pasta primavera (pasta, broccoli, carrots, onion, peas, olive oil, Parmesan)	8 oz	425	20	42

	AMOUNT	CALORIES	FAT-GRAMS	% FAT
in cream sauce	12 oz	1,200	75	56
w/ chicken	8 oz	475	20	38
w/ ham	8 oz	475	23	43
w/ salami (pasta, cauliflower, zucchini, sweet peppers, onion, olive oil, salami, Parmesan)	8 oz	520	35	60
Pasta quattroformaggi (w/ four cheeses: Gorgonzola, mozzarella, Gruyère, Parmesan)	1 cup	540	31	52
Pastitsio (pasta, ground lamb, tomato sauce, egg sauce, Parmesan)	10 oz	605	41	61
Penne all'Arrabiata (pasta, spicy tomato sauce, pancetta)	10 oz	490	15	28
Ravioli (10 spinach ravioli, 6 oz sauce)				
w/ Alfredo sauce	1 serving	1,165	51	40
w/ red sauce	1 serving	630	15	21
w/ tomato meat sauce	1 serving	740	23	28
Shells:				
Baked shells (Fontina cheese, shrimp)	10 oz	450	21	42

	AMOUNT	CALORIES	FAT-GRAMS	% FAT
Seafood-stuffed shells (ricotta, milk, celery, zucchini, onion, shrimp, crab)	3 shells	300	6	18
Shells w/ white clam sauce	9 oz	455	6	12
Spaetzle	4 oz	275	10	32
Tortellini:				
& vegetable confetti	9 oz	435	23	48
w/ Alfredo sauce (10 spinach tortellini, 6 oz sauce)	1 serving	1,165	51	40
w/ red sauce (10 spinach tortellini, 6 oz sauce)	1 serving	630	15	21
w/ tomato/meat sauce (10 spinach tortellini, 6 oz sauce)	1 serving	740	23	28
Vermicelli Ballerini (pasta, olive oil, walnuts, powdered sugar, nutmeg, allspice)	6 oz	880	26	26

PIZZA

	AMOUNT	CALORIES	FAT-GRAMS	% FAT
Calzone:				
Mushroom & prosciutto	1	540	25	42
Sausage & mushroom	1	520	25	43
Pizza:				
Pesto pizza	1 slice of 7" pie	500	32	57
Pizza alla Napoletana (tomato-cheese pizza)	1 slice of 7" pie	305	14	41
White pizza	⅙ of 12" pie	365	16	39
Pizza add-ons:				
Artichoke hearts	1 oz	30	2	60
Black olives	1 oz	30	3	90
Canadian bacon	1 oz	45	2	40
Green peppers	1 oz	5	0	0
Ground beef	1 oz	80	6	67
Italian sausage	1 oz	90	8	80
Jalapeño peppers	1 oz	10	0	0
Mushrooms	1 oz	10	0	0

	AMOUNT	CALORIES	FAT-GRAMS	% FAT
Onions	1 oz	10	0	0
Pepperoni	1 oz	140	13	84
Pineapple tidbits	½ cup	50	0	0
Salami	1 oz	110	10	82

POULTRY & POULTRY DISHES

	AMOUNT	CALORIES	FAT-GRAMS	% FAT
CHICKEN				
Arroz con pollo	I serving	515	25	43
Baked chicken	I quarter	340	22	58
Greek-style				
(w/ potatoes, onions,				
lemon sauce)	I quarter	575	30	47
w/ orzo (1 cup)	I quarter	645	35	49
Batter-fried chicken	I quarter	455	27	53
BBQ chicken	I quarter	405	25	56
BBQ chicken burger				
(grilled chicken,				
lettuce, tomato, onion,				
& BBQ sauce on bun)	I	320	6	17
BBQ chicken burger				
deluxe (grilled				
chicken, lettuce,				
tomato, onion,				
BBQ sauce, cheese				
& mayo on bun)	I	495	22	40
Blackened chicken	½ breast	285	17	54
Black mushroom				
chicken	main dish	295	15	46
Boiled chicken	I quarter	240	9	34

	AMOUNT	CALORIES	FAT-GRAMS	% FAT
Border chicken burger (grilled chicken, cheese, green chilies, tomatoes & guacamole on hard roll)	1	965	68	53
Broiled chicken, spicy hot	1 half	665	41	55
Brunswick stew	10 oz	315	13	37
Cajun chicken	4 oz	285	17	54
Chicken à la king	6 oz	225	13	51
Chicken & chips	1 serving	400	22	51
Chicken & dumpling (1 pc chicken, 1 dumpling, sauce)	main dish	375	23	55
Chicken & peppers (½ breast w/ peppers)	1 serving	225	10	40
Chicken & rice casserole	8 oz	280	7	22
Chicken breast fillet w/ skin	½ breast	195	8	37
w/o skin	½ breast	140	3	21
Chicken breast sandwich (w/ mayo & lettuce)	1	355	19	48
Chicken breast w/ prosciutto & fontina	½ breast	245	12	44
Chicken burgoo	10 oz	495	16	29
Chicken Cacciatore	10 oz	250	13	46
Chicken Caesar wrap	1	630	31	44
Chicken Calvados	½ breast	305	19	56
Chicken club sandwich	1	545	26	43
Chicken Cordon Bleu	1 breast	800	50	56

	AMOUNT	CALORIES	FAT-GRAMS	% FAT
Chicken Creole	8 oz	275	11	36
Chicken crepes w/ cream sauce	2	875	51	52
Chicken croquettes (2 oz each)	2	350	16	41
Chicken curry	6 oz	255	15	52
Chicken Diavolo (breaded chicken breast, Parmesan, Dijon sauce)	main dish	625	28	40
Chicken Dijon (w/ 2 oz Dijon cream sauce)	½ breast	405	17	37
Chicken Divan	6 oz	385	18	42
Chicken fajita roll-up	1	705	36	43
Chicken fricassee	6 oz	260	16	56
Chicken gumbo	8 oz	125	5	36
Chicken hash	1 cup	240	11	41
Chicken hot dog Regular	1	115	9	70
Jumbo	1	290	26	81
Chicken Jack Daniel's	½ breast	300	19	56
Chicken Jambalaya	8 oz	340	12	32
Chicken kabobs	1 kabob	273	10	33
Chicken Kiev	1 breast	730	42	52
Chicken liver sauté	6 oz	255	14	49
Chicken livers hunter-style (w/ tomatoes, tomato paste, mushrooms, onions)	6 oz	260	14	48

	AMOUNT	CALORIES	FAT-GRAMS	% FAT
Chicken loaf				
w/ fricassee sauce	6 oz	380	20	47
Chicken Lorraine				
(w/ mushrooms,				
artichokes, cream				
sauce)	1 breast	775	50	58
Chicken Marsala	4 oz	445	26	52
Chicken Nogada				
(chicken breast,				
almonds, mushrooms,				
sauce)	4 oz	530	40	68
Chicken nuggets	½ breast	775	50	58
Chicken Oscar	4 oz	870	67	69
Chicken paprika				
w/ noodles (1 quarter				
chicken, 3 oz				
noodles/sauce)	1 serving	595	28	42
Chicken paprikash				
(chicken, sour cream				
sauce)	1 quarter	455	30	59
Chicken Parmigiana	1 breast	625	28	40
Chicken pasta				
primavera	1½ cups	290	12	37
Chicken patties				
(½ breast w/o skin)				
Fried	1 serving	290	19	59
Grilled	1 serving	140	3	19
Chicken piccata	4 oz	415	25	54
Chicken pilaf (1 quarter				
chicken, 8 oz pilaf)	1 serving	715	44	55

	AMOUNT	CALORIES	FAT-GRAMS	% FAT
Chicken Polynesian (w/ vegetables, sweet & sour sauce)	8 oz	285	17	54
Chicken Portugal (marinated in olive oil, grilled)	4 oz	290	19	59
Chicken pot pie	8 oz	800	60	67
Chicken Royal Hawaiian (w/ mushrooms, almonds, coconut)	6 oz	400	27	60
Chicken saltimbocca	1 breast	800	50	56
Chicken pocket sandwich (chicken, lettuce & tomato in pita)	1	255	3	10
Chicken salad sandwich	1	335	17	56
Chicken sandwich deluxe (chicken, lettuce, tomato, garlic, feta cheese, onion & olive oil in pita)	1	395	25	57
Chicken soufflé	5½ oz	295	19	58
Chicken stew	10 oz	315	13	37
Chicken-stuffed baked tomato	2 halves	255	12	42
Chicken tetrazzini	8 oz	460	18	35
Chicken w/ black bean sauce	6 oz	320	18	51
Chicken w/ olives & pine nuts	3 oz	285	18	57

	AMOUNT	CALORIES	FAT-GRAMS	% FAT
Coq au vin	1 quarter	505	35	62
Coq au vin sauté	½ breast	315	11	31
Crab-filled breast of chicken w/ Hollandaise sauce	1 pc	735	67	82
Creamed chicken	6 oz	275	16	52
& ham on corn bread	8 oz	560	27	44
& vegetables on biscuit	6 oz	445	24	48
Escalloped chicken & noodles	8 oz	315	14	40
Fried chicken	2 pcs	525	28	48
Garlic chicken	main dish	365	10	25
Ginger chicken	main dish	375	10	24
Green pepper chicken	main dish	296	15	46
Lemon chicken (3 oz grilled breast, 2 oz lemon sauce)	1 serving	290	14	43
Malibu chicken (1 breast, ham, cheese, mustard sauce)	main dish	800	50	56
Mediterranean chicken wrap	1	580	22	34
Mesquite grilled chicken (½ breast w/o skin, basted w/ olive oil)	1 serving	215	5	22
Mexican-style chicken: Chimichanga (chicken, cheese, tortilla, sour cream)	1	605	35	52

	AMOUNT	CALORIES	FAT-GRAMS	% FAT
Enchilada w/ sour cream sauce	1	575	33	52
Enchilada verde & sour cream	1	450	30	60
Fajita (chicken, peppers, onion, tortilla)	1	415	21	45
w/ cheese, guacamole & sour cream	1	780	44	51
Flauta (tortilla, chicken filling)	1	225	10	40
Quesadilla	1	375	17	41
Sopito (chicken, lettuce, tomato, cheese)	1	435	21	44
Taco w/ cheese, avocado & salsa	1	435	21	44
Tostada (chicken, beans, cheese, olives, avocado, sour cream)	1	935	55	52
Paella	main dish	675	28	37
Pine nut chicken (w/ brandy cream sauce)	4 oz	530	40	68
Roast chicken w/ new potatoes	1 quarter	550	28	46
Roast chicken w/ rosemary	4 oz	285	10	34
Rotisserie chicken	1 half	665	41	55
Smothered chicken (w/ onion, mushrooms, cream sauce)	½ breast	775	50	58

	AMOUNT	CALORIES	FAT-GRAMS	% FAT
Snow White chicken	main dish	295	15	46
Southwestern chicken wrap	1	795	41	46
Stuffed chicken breast (bread stuffing, sauce)	1 breast	395	26	59
Oriental-style chicken:				
Almond chicken	main dish	580	38	59
Cashew chicken	main dish	580	36	57
Chicken & snow peas	main dish	295	15	46
Chicken chop suey	8 oz	185	8	38
Chicken chow mein	6 oz	180	8	40
Chicken teriyaki	1 quarter	355	17	43
Hot & sour chicken	main dish	300	15	45
Kung Pao chicken	8 oz	490	25	46
Stir-fried chicken				
w/ eggplant	main dish	385	20	46
w/ vegetables	6 oz	245	14	51
Sweet & sour chicken	8 oz	305	6	18
Thai-style chicken	main dish	320	17	48
CORNISH GAME HEN				
Baked Cornish game hen	½ hen	400	25	56
Orange-glazed Cornish game hen w/ wild rice stuffing	1 bird	560	26	42
DUCK				
Roast duck à l'orange	1 quarter	835	69	75
	1 half	1,745	139	72
Szechuan duck	1 half	1,285	108	75

	AMOUNT	CALORIES	FAT-GRAMS	% FAT
GOOSE				
Roast goose	6 oz	360	25	63
Roast goose Provençal	9 oz	730	48	59
PHEASANT				
Roast pheasant w/ sausage dressing	1 quarter	1,105	69	56
Roast pheasant w/ wild rice dressing (8 oz pheasant, ½ cup dressing)	1 serving	860	44	46
QUAIL				
Roast quail (4 oz quail)	2 birds	500	36	65
TURKEY				
Baked turkey legs	1 leg	420	13	30
Cranberry-sauced turkey steaks	4 oz	255	8	28
Grilled turkey piccata	6 oz	265	9	31
Hot turkey sandwich w/ gravy	1	410	10	22
Roast turkey	6 oz	385	18	42
Turkey & biscuit	6 oz	395	20	46
Turkey & cream cheese sandwich w/ cranberry chutney	1	470	28	54
Turkey breast sandwich w/ mayo	1	420	18	39
w/o mayo	1	380	7	20

	AMOUNT	CALORIES	FAT-GRAMS	% FAT
Turkey club sandwich w/ bacon & tomato				
w/ mayo	1	850	34	36
w/o mayo	1	750	23	25
Turkey Divan	8 oz	630	33	47
Turkey fillet burger deluxe (grilled turkey, bacon, tomato & cheese on bread)	1	445	25	50
Turkey gumbo	8 oz	95	4	38
Turkey loaf				
Breast meat	4 oz	125	2	15
Light & dark meat	4 oz	225	13	52
Turkey meatballs (1" each)	3	325	14	38
Turkey mole	10 oz	530	26	44
Turkey patties, breaded & fried	1	180	12	60
Turkey wings Creole	1 wing	450	6	21
Scalloped turkey	8 oz	255	6	21

RICE & OTHER GRAINS

	AMOUNT	CALORIES	FAT-GRAMS	% FAT
Barley w/ mushrooms	3 oz	180	5	25
Bulgur w/ Parmesan	⅔ cup	190	3	13
Chop suey:				
w/ chicken	8 oz	255	10	35
w/ pork	8 oz	195	10	46
Corn fritters				
(1.5 oz each)	2	120	3	23
Cornmeal:				
Fried polenta (2 oz each)	2 slices	295	16	49
Hamburger & rice				
casserole	1 cup	375	21	50
Hush puppies				
(1.5 oz each)	2	140	5	32
Couscous (no fat added)	⅔ cup	110	1	7
Dressings/stuffings:				
Bread (½ cup)	3 oz	290	12	37
Chestnut	3 oz	225	11	44
Corn bread	3 oz	240	12	45
& sausage	4 oz	250	17	61
Oyster corn bread	3 oz	185	11	53
Sausage	3 oz	260	9	31
Wild rice	4 oz	115	3	23
Dumpling (1.5 oz)	1	115	3	23

	AMOUNT	CALORIES	FAT-GRAMS	% FAT
Grits:				
No fat added	1 cup	145	0	0
w/ 2 tsp butter	1 cup	225	8	72
Grits au gratin	½ cup	190	12	56
Matzo cakes				
(w/ olive oil)	4 oz	250	20	72
Polenta:				
Baked polenta				
(w/ fontina,				
Gorgonzola)	1 slice	625	32	46
Soft polenta				
w/ bacon &				
rosemary	1 serving	185	8	38
w/ sausage	1 serving	360	16	40
Rice:				
Baked rice	side dish	330	13	35
Browned rice	3 oz	160	5	28
Cajun dirty rice	1½ cup	315	19	54
Cheese rice				
croquettes				
(3 oz each)	2	520	23	40
Curried rice	3 oz	150	6	36
Fried rice	3 oz	140	4	26
Herbed rice				
(no fat added)	3 oz	110	1	8
Maui rice	8 oz	395	15	34
Rice & bean sprouts	1 cup	295	7	21
Rice & mushrooms	3 oz	130	5	34
Rice Calcutta	3 oz	105	3	25
Rice, peas & pancetta	5 oz	380	10	24

	AMOUNT	CALORIES	FAT-GRAMS	% FAT
Rice pilaf	3 oz	150	6	36
Greek-style	6 oz	330	10	27
Turkish-style (w/ pine nuts & almonds)	6 oz	420	20	43
Rice pilaf & spinach	12 oz	310	11	32
Tomato fried rice	4 oz	170	9	48
Risotto:				
Risotto primavera	10 oz	460	20	39
Wild mushroom risotto	6 oz	395	15	34
Saffron rice	3 oz	150	6	30
Spanish rice	4 oz	115	3	23
White rice (w/ ½ tsp butter)	3 oz	115	2	15
Wild rice casserole	3 oz	125	5	36

RICE/OTHER GRAINS

SALADS & SALAD DRESSINGS

	AMOUNT	CALORIES	FAT-GRAMS	% FAT
SALADS				
(Dressing included unless otherwise noted)				
Ambrosia fruit salad	side dish	215	2	8
Antipasto platter	side dish	230	15	59
Apple & date salad	1 cup	310	19	55
Apple & grape salad	1 cup	265	19	64
Apple-grape aspic w/ walnuts	5 oz	140	4	25
Apricot, banana & grape salad (no dressing)	1 cup	85	0	0
Apricot parfait salad	1 serving	185	9	44
Artichoke, avocado & orange salad	1 artichoke	300	20	60
Asparagus vinaigrette	3 spears	60	6	77
Asparagus & egg	side dish	205	16	70
Asparagus & tomato salad	side dish	125	10	73
Avocado, tomato & chicken salad (no dressing)	1 cup	175	9	47
Banana-berry salad	side dish	110	0	0

	AMOUNT	CALORIES	FAT-GRAMS	% FAT
Beef salads:				
Beef & apple salad	main dish	345	19	49
Beef & broccoli salad	main dish	310	21	61
Beef & fruit salad	main dish	400	24	54
Beef vegetable stir-fry salad	main dish	240	12	45
Beef, pasta & bean salad	main dish	365	13	32
Beef salad w/ vegetables	1.5 cup	255	14	49
Marinated steak salad w/ shiitake mushrooms	main dish	325	23	63
Pasta, beef & vegetable salad	main dish	525	34	58
Steak salad	main dish	330	21	57
Taco salad	1.5 cup	455	37	73
Belgian endive salad	1 head	205	21	57
Broccoli & egg salad	side dish	340	30	80
Broccoli & tomato salad	side dish	265	24	82
Cabbage, carrots & green pepper salad (no dressing)	1 cup	35	0	0
Caesar salad	main dish	415	40	86
Cardinal salad (3" × 3")	1 serving	100	0	0
Carrot, apple & raisin salad	1 cup	390	28	64
Carrot, pineapple & raisin salad	1 cup	405	29	71

	AMOUNT	CALORIES	FAT-GRAMS	% FAT
Cauliflower & tomato salad	side dish	270	23	77
Chef's salad bowl (no dressing)	1.5 cup	365	32	79
Cherry crunch salad (3" × 3")	1 serving	185	2	10
Chicken salads:				
Chicken almond salad	1 cup	385	32	75
Chicken & pasta salad	main dish	455	23	45
Chicken artichoke salad	main dish	410	26	57
Chicken, avocado & tomato (no dressing)	1.5 cup	175	9	47
Chicken Caesar salad	main dish	550	48	78
Chicken fajita salad	main dish	365	14	34
w/ 1 tbsp guacamole	add	50	6	100
w/ 1 tbsp sour cram	add	25	3	100
w/ 1 tbsp tomato salsa	add	5	0	0
Chicken-filled melon (no dressing)	main dish	250	4	14
Chicken salad "Fat Watcher"	main dish	240	5	19
Chicken salad w/ tortellini & sun-dried tomatoes	main dish	510	20	35
Chicken salad w/ wild rice	main dish	430	19	40
Chicken spinach salad	main dish	370	27	65
w/ chutney	main dish	460	28	55
Chicken taco salad	main dish	425	26	55

	AMOUNT	CALORIES	FAT-GRAMS	% FAT
Curried chicken cashew salad	main dish	625	45	65
Fried chicken & spinach salad	main dish	370	27	65
Grilled chicken & vegetable salad (no dressing)	main dish	245	9	33
Grilled chicken Waldorf salad	main dish	460	28	55
Hot chicken salad w/ honey mustard dressing	main dish	505	34	60
Peking chicken salad (no dressing)	main dish	230	7	27
Sesame chicken & rice salad	main dish	330	15	41
Stir-fry chicken salad (no dressing)	main dish	410	34	74
Thai chicken salad (no dressing)	main dish	310	6	18
Tomato stuffed w/ chicken salad	1	265	17	58
Chinese cabbage salad	1 cup	210	13	56
Cobb salad	main dish	495	36	65
Coleslaw	1 cup	210	13	56
Cottage cheese & chives	½ cup	115	5	39
Cottage cheese & fruit	1 serving	195	5	23
Cottage cheese & vegetables	¼ cup	45	2	38
Couscous salad	side dish	275	15	49

	AMOUNT	CALORIES	FAT-GRAMS	% FAT
Crab Louie	main dish	590	47	71
Crab salad w/ melon	main dish	360	23	57
Cucumber & onion salad	1 cup	165	14	76
Cucumber-lime salad, molded (3" × 3")	1 serving	80	2	22
Cucumbers in sour cream	1 cup	135	9	60
Curried chicken cashew salad	main dish	625	45	65
Duck salad	main dish	450	32	64
w/ fruit		640	41	58
Fajita salad	main dish	365	14	34
w/ 1 tbsp guacamole	*add*	50	6	100
w/ 1 tbsp sour cream	*add*	25	3	100
w/ 1 tbsp tomato salsa	*add*	5	0	0
Fried chicken & spinach salad	main dish	370	27	65
Fruit salads:				
Ambrosia fruit salad	side dish	215	2	8
Apple & date salad	1 cup	310	19	55
Apple & grape salad	1 cup	265	19	64
Apple-grape aspic w/ walnuts	5 oz	140	4	25
Apricot, banana & grape salad (no dressing)	1 cup	85	0	0
Apricot parfait salad	1 serving	185	9	44
Artichoke, avocado & orange salad	1 artichoke	300	20	60
Avocado, orange & grapefruit salad	side dish	340	31	82

	AMOUNT	CALORIES	FAT-GRAMS	% FAT
Banana-berry salad	side dish	110	0	0
Beef & apple salad	main dish	345	19	49
Beef & fruit salad	main dish	400	24	54
Carrot & raisin salad	1 cup	375	28	67
Carrot, apple & raisin salad	1 cup	390	28	64
Carrot, pineapple & raisin salad	1 cup	405	29	71
Cherry crunch salad (3" × 3")	1 serving	185	2	10
Chicken-filled melons (no dressing)	main dish	250	4	14
Cottage cheese & fruit	1 serving	195	5	23
Cucumber-lime salad (3" × 3")	1 serving	80	2	22
Crab salad w/ melon	main dish	360	23	57
Duck salad w/ fruit	main dish	640	41	58
Fruit & cream cheese	½ cup	170	4	21
Fruit marshmallow	½ cup	120	4	30
Fruit plate (fruit only)	side dish	230	0	0
Fruit platter w/ 1 oz cheese wedge	1 serving	320	10	28
Fruit salad				
w/ avocado	1 serving	300	16	48
w/ cottage cheese	1 serving	195	5	23
w/ creamy dressing	1 cup	245	18	67
Grapefruit basket	1 serving	190	0	0
Grapefruit salad	½ cup	76	0	0

	AMOUNT	CALORIES	FAT-GRAMS	% FAT
Grilled chicken Waldorf salad	main dish	460	28	55
Hazelnut, pear & arugula salad	side dish	110	9	73
Jellied cranberry & apple	½ cup	205	0	0
Jellied cranberry relish	½ cup	205	0	0
Lime-pear aspic (3" × 3")	1 serving	95	0	0
Lobster-melon salad	main dish	375	20	48
Melon salad	1 cup	55	0	0
Molded fruit salads *See* Molded salads				
Peach half stuffed w/ cream cheese	1 serving	95	3	29
Pineapple boat fruit salad	1 serving	255	0	0
Pineapple-lime salad	½ cup	145	7	41
Pineapple ring & stuffed dates	1 serving	60	3	44
Regal fruit salad w/ whipped topping	½ cup	150	7	41
Ribbon mold	½ cup	290	16	50
Scallop salad w/ fruit salsa (no dressing)	side dish	120	1	7
Spinach chutney salad	main dish	460	28	55
Summer fruit salad	1 cup	90	0	0
Tropical fruit salad	1 cup	100	0	0
Tropical fruits w/ lime syrup	1 cup	120	0	0

	AMOUNT	CALORIES	FAT-GRAMS	% FAT
Waldorf salad	1 cup	255	15	52
Waldorf salad mold	½ cup	135	4	26
Winter fruit salad	1 cup	115	0	0
Gado-gado	side dish	280	21	68
Garden primavera salad				
(no dressing)	1 cup	15	0	0
Grapefruit basket	1 serving	190	0	0
Grapefruit salad	½ cup	76	0	0
Greek salad	side dish	280	21	68
Greek-style pasta salad	main dish	405	30	66
Green salad	1 cup	150	15	89
w/ fresh basil,				
mozzarella, tomato				
(no dressing)	side dish	270	15	50
w/ chèvre				
(goat cheese)	side dish	345	26	68
Grilled chicken &				
vegetable salad				
(no dressing)	main dish	245	9	33
Grilled chicken				
Waldorf salad	main dish	460	28	55
Grilled swordfish salad				
(w/ olives, onion,				
oranges, arugula)	main dish	450	31	65
Ham & cheese platter				
w/ potato salad	side dish	390	24	56
Ham & rice salad	1 cup	370	10	24
Ham salad platter				
w/ potato chips	1 serving	595	45	68
Hearts of palm salad	side dish	95	7	66

	AMOUNT	CALORIES	FAT-GRAMS	% FAT
Hot chicken salad w/ honey mustard dressing	main dish	505	34	60
Hot curried pork salad	main dish	410	25	55
Jellied cranberry & apple	½ cup	205	0	0
Jellied cranberry relish	½ cup	205	0	0
Jellied fruit	½ cup	100	0	0
Lamb brochette salad	main dish	465	26	50
Layered 24-hour salad	side dish	365	35	86
Lime-pear aspic (3" × 3")	1 serving	95	0	0
Lobster-melon salad	main dish	375	20	48
Macaroni & ham salad	1 cup	390	22	51
Macaroni salad	1 cup	360	18	45
Marinated broccoli	side dish	110	10	82
Marinated cauliflower	½ cup	110	10	83
Marinated cucumber salad	½ cup	115	9	70
Marinated green bean salad	side dish	205	20	88
Marinated mixed vegetable salad	1 cup	230	17	74
Marinated mushroom salad	side dish	90	7	71
Marinated steak salad w/ shiitake mushrooms	main dish	330	23	63
Marinated vegetable & cheese salad	side dish	255	24	85
Melon salad	1 cup	55	0	0

	AMOUNT	CALORIES	FAT-GRAMS	% FAT
Molded salads:				
Apple-grape aspic w/ walnuts	5 oz	140	4	25
Apricot parfait salad	1 serving	185	9	44
Cardinal salad (3" × 3")	1 serving	10	0	0
Cherry crunch salad (3" × 3")	1 serving	185	2	10
Cucumber-lime salad (3" × 3")	1 serving	80	2	22
Fruit & cream cheese	½ cup	170	4	21
Fruit marshmallow	½ cup	120	4	30
Jellied cranberry & apple	½ cup	205	0	0
Jellied fruit	½ cup	205	0	0
Lime-pear aspic (3" × 3")	1 serving	95	0	0
Molded Bing cherry salad w/ walnuts	½ cup	145	4	25
Molded citrus salad	1 serving	95	0	0
Molded creamy lime salad	½ cup	160	6	34
Molded mandarin orange salad	5 oz	95	0	0
Perfection salad	½ cup	105	0	0
Pineapple-lime salad	½ cup	145	7	43
Regal fruit salad w/ whipped topping	½ cup	150	7	41
Ribbon mold	½ cup	290	16	50
Seafood aspic	½ cup	70	1	13

	AMOUNT	CALORIES	FAT-GRAMS	% FAT
Tomato aspic	½ cup	35	0	0
Tuna mousse	½ cup	280	19	61
Waldorf salad mold	½ cup	135	4	26
Oriental noodle salad	main dish	300	8	24
Oriental salad	side dish	210	15	65
Pasta salads:				
Beef, pasta & bean salad	main dish	365	13	32
Chicken & pasta salad	side dish	455	23	45
Greek-style pasta salad	main dish	405	30	66
Macaroni & ham salad	1 cup	390	22	51
Macaroni salad	1 cup	360	18	45
Oriental noodle salad	main dish	300	8	24
Pasta & bean salad	side dish	270	16	53
Pasta & salami salad	main dish	670	52	70
Pasta & shrimp salad	main dish	480	24	45
Pasta, beef & vegetable salad	main dish	530	34	58
Pasta, ham & cheese salad	main dish	490	25	46
Pasta primavera salad	1 cup	365	27	67
Pasta salad	1 cup	360	18	45
Peking chicken salad (no dressing)	main dish	230	7	27
Pesto pasta salad	1 cup	400	26	58
Salmon & pasta salad	main dish	485	31	57
Seafood pasta salad	main dish	480	24	45
Tortellini salad	main dish	580	40	62

	AMOUNT	CALORIES	FAT-GRAMS	% FAT
Tortellini shrimp salad	main dish	560	32	51
Trio salad platter	main dish	675	46	61
Turkey & vegetable salad	main dish	420	22	47
Turkey, black bean & pasta salad	main dish	570	30	47
Peach half stuffed w/ cream cheese	1 serving	93	3	29
Peking chicken salad (no dressing)	main dish	230	7	27
Perfection salad	½ cup	105	0	0
Pesto pasta salad	1 cup	400	26	58
Pickled beets w/ egg slices		135	3	20
w/ onions		105	0	0
Pineapple fruit boat salad	1 serving	255	0	0
Pineapple-lime salad	½ cup	145	7	43
Pineapple ring & stuffed dates	1 serving	60	3	44
Poached salmon & marinated vegetable platter	main dish	470	33	63
Pork salads:				
Chef's salad bowl (no dressing)	1.5 cup	365	32	79
Ham & cheese platter	1 serving	390	24	56
Ham & rice salad	1 cup	370	10	24
Ham salad platter w/ potato chips	1 serving	595	45	68

	AMOUNT	CALORIES	FAT-GRAMS	% FAT
Hot curried pork salad	main dish	410	25	55
Macaroni & ham salad	1 cup	390	22	51
Pasta, ham & cheese salad	main dish	490	25	46
Pork & cabbage salad	main dish	545	26	43
Pork & roasted pepper salad	main dish	310	23	66
Potato salads:				
Hot German potato salad	1 cup	250	16	58
Old-fashioned potato salad	1 cup	300	18	54
Potato salad w/ sliced Polish sausage (½ cup salad, 3 oz sausage)	1 serving	395	26	59
Salami-potato salad plate	main dish	640	43	60
Seafood & potato salad	main dish	485	29	54
Regal fruit salad w/ whipped topping	½ cup	150	7	41
Relish plate	1 serving	50	1	17
Ribbon mold	½ cup	290	16	50
Rice & avocado salad	side dish	285	20	64
Rice & vegetable salad	1 cup	305	17	50
Roasted pepper salad	side dish	75	5	58
Roasted pepper, tomato & olive salad	side dish	295	25	76

	AMOUNT	CALORIES	FAT-GRAMS	% FAT
Salami & pasta salad	main dish	670	52	70
Salami-potato salad plate	main dish	640	43	60
Salmon salads:				
Poached salmon & marinated vegetable platter	main dish	470	33	63
Salmon & pasta salad	main dish	485	31	57
Salmon & potato salad	main dish	615	40	59
Salmon salad	side dish	235	11	42
Smoked salmon platter	1 serving	240	9	34
Scallop salad w/ fruit salsa (no dressing)	side dish	120	1	7
Seafood salads:				
Crab Louie	main dish	590	47	71
Crab salad w/ melon	main dish	360	23	57
Grilled swordfish salad (w/ olives, onion, oranges, arugula)	main dish	450	31	65
Lobster-melon salad	main dish	375	20	48
Pasta & shrimp salad	main dish	480	24	45
Scallop salad w/ fruit salsa (no dressing)	main dish	120	1	7
Seafood & potato salad	main dish	485	29	54
Seafood aspic	½ cup	70	1	13

	AMOUNT	CALORIES	FAT GRAMS	% FAT
Seafood pasta salad	main dish	480	24	45
Seafood salad	main dish	650	49	68
Seviche salad	main dish	200	11	50
Shrimp bowl (no dressing)	side dish	120	3	22
Shrimp Caesar salad	main dish	535	42	70
Shrimp Louie	1 serving	590	47	71
Shrimp salad Oriental-style	main dish	260	15	52
Shrimp salad sushi-style (no dressing)	main dish	195	2	10
Shrimp taco salad	main dish	650	49	68
Sole salad w/ asparagus & mixed greens	side dish	300	19	57
Tomato stuffed w/ tuna salad	1	175	11	56
Tortellini shrimp salad	main dish	560	32	51
Trio salad platter	main dish	675	46	61
Tuna fish & mixed vegetable salad	1 serving	425	32	67
Tuna fish chef's salad bowl (no dressing)	1.5 cup	345	31	81
Tuna-havarti salad	main dish	380	26	61
Tuna mousse	½ cup	280	19	61
Warm tuna salad	main dish	250	10	36
Wild rice & shrimp salad	main dish	260	15	52

	AMOUNT	CALORIES	FAT-GRAMS	% FAT
Sesame chicken & rice salad	main dish	330	15	41
Seviche salad	main dish	200	11	50
Shrimp salads:				
Pasta & shrimp salad	main dish	480	24	45
Shrimp bowl (no dressing)	side dish	120	3	22
Shrimp Caesar salad	main dish	535	42	70
Shrimp Louie	1 serving	590	47	71
Shrimp salad Oriental-style	main dish	260	15	52
Shrimp salad sushi-style (no dressing)	main dish	195	2	10
Shrimp taco salad	main dish	650	49	68
Tortellini shrimp salad	main dish	560	32	51
Wild rice & shrimp salad	main dish	260	15	52
Sole salad w/ asparagus & mixed greens	side dish	300	19	57
Spinach-chutney salad	main dish	460	28	55
Spinach salad (no dressing)	1 cup	255	6	21
w/ chicken (no dressing)	main dish	370	27	65
Steak salad	main dish	330	21	57
Stir-fry chicken salad	main dish	410	34	74
Stuffed head of lettuce	side dish	110	10	92
Summer fruit salad	1 cup	90	0	0
Tabbouleh salad	side dish	245	14	51

	AMOUNT	CALORIES	FAT-GRAMS	% FAT
Taco salad	1.5 cup	455	37	73
w/ tostada shell		50	2	36
per ½ fresh avocado	add	155	14	82
per 1 tbsp guacamole	add	50	6	100
per 1 tbsp salsa	add	5	0	0
per 1 tbsp sour cream	add	25	3	100
Thai chicken salad				
(no dressing)	main dish	310	6	18
Three-bean salad	1 cup	310	14	41
Tomato salads:				
Asparagus & tomato				
salad	side dish	125	10	73
Avocado, tomato &				
chicken salad				
(no dressing)	main dish	175	9	47
Broccoli & tomato				
salad	side dish	265	24	82
Cauliflower & tomato				
salad	side dish	270	23	77
Chicken, avocado &				
tomato (no dressing)	1.5 cup	175	9	47
Chicken salad				
w/ tortellini &				
sun-dried tomatoes	main dish	510	20	35
Green salad w/ fresh				
basil, mozzarella				
& tomato	side dish	270	15	50
Tomato à l'Andalouse	1 tomato	230	22	86
Tomato & avocado				
(no dressing)	side dish	90	8	78

	AMOUNT	CALORIES	FAT-GRAMS	% FAT
Tomato & cucumber (no dressing)	side dish	25	0	0
Tomato & green pepper rings (no dressing)	side dish	20	0	0
Tomato & onion salad	1 cup	160	13	72
Tomato aspic	½ cup	35	0	0
Tomato stuffed	½ cup	80	6	67
Tomato stuffed w/ chicken salad	1	265	17	58
Tomato stuffed w/ tuna salad	1	175	11	56
Tortellini salad	side dish	290	20	62
Tortellini shrimp salad	main dish	560	32	51
Tossed green salad (no dressing)	1 cup	15	0	0
Tossed greens w/ nasturtiums	side dish	115	11	85
Trio salad platter	main dish	675	46	61
Tropical fruit salad	1 cup	100	0	0
Tropical fruits w/ lime syrup	1 cup	120	0	0
Tuna fish & mixed vegetable salad	1 serving	425	32	67
Tuna fish chef's salad bowl (no dressing)	1.5 cup	345	31	81
Tuna-havarti salad	main dish	380	26	61
Tuna mousse	½ cup	280	19	61
Turkey & vegetable salad	main dish	420	22	47

	AMOUNT	CALORIES	FAT-GRAMS	% FAT
Turkey, black bean & pasta salad	main dish	570	30	47
Turkey cold platter (no dressing)	main dish	375	6	19
Vegetable salad (no dressing)	1 cup	15	0	0
Vegetable salad à la Russe	1 cup	290	22	68
Vegetable tray	2 oz	40	0	0
Waldorf salad	1 cup	255	15	52
Waldorf salad mold	½ cup	135	4	26
Warm tuna salad	main dish	250	10	36
Wild rice & shrimp salad	main dish	260	15	52
Wilted greens salad w/ bacon dressing	1 cup	255	28	99
Winter fruit salad (no dressing)	1 cup	115	0	0
SALAD BAR ADD-ONS				
Alfalfa sprouts	1 oz	10	0	0
American cheese	1 oz	105	9	75
Applesauce	1 cup	100	0	0
Bacon bits	½ oz	40	2	45
Banana chips	1 oz	100	0	0
Beets	1 cup	60	0	0
Blueberries	1 tbsp	5	0	0
Bread sticks	2	35	1	28
Broccoli	½ cup	15	0	0
Cabbage	1 cup	15	0	0

	AMOUNT	CALORIES	FAT-GRAMS	% FAT
Cantaloupe	2 pcs	15	0	0
Carrots	¼ cup	10	0	0
Cauliflower	½ cup	15	0	0
Cheddar cheese	1 oz	115	9	71
Cherry peppers	1 tbsp	5	0	0
Chow mein noodles	1 oz	140	6	38
Coconut	1 oz	160	11	62
Coleslaw	3.5 oz	70	4	51
Cottage cheese	½ cup	125	5	35
Crackers (saltines)	2	25	1	36
Croutons	½ oz	70	3	38
Cucumbers	4 slices	5	0	0
Eggs	1 egg	80	5	56
Garbanzo beans	½ cup	360	5	12
Gelatin				
Lime	½ cup	90	0	0
Strawberry	½ cup	90	0	0
Grapefruit sections	1 cup	80	0	0
Grapes	1 cup	100	0	0
Green peppers	¼ cup	10	0	0
Honeydew melon	2 pcs	25	0	0
Jalapeño peppers	1 tbsp	10	0	0
Kale	1 oz	15	0	0
Kidney beans	¼ cup	55	0	0
Lettuce	2 leaves	5	0	0
Macaroni salad	½ cup	150	9	54
Mozzarella	1 oz	90	7	70
Part skim	1 oz	70	5	64
Mushrooms	¼ cup	5	0	0
Oil	1 tbsp	120	14	100

	AMOUNT	CALORIES	FAT-GRAMS	% FAT
Onions	¼ cup	10	0	0
Oranges	2 oz	25	0	0
Pasta salad	½ cup	180	9	45
Parmesan, grated	1 tbsp	25	2	78
Peaches	2 slices	15	0	0
Peas	1 oz	25	0	0
Pepper rings, pickled	1 tbsp	5	0	0
Pickle spear	1	10	0	0
Pineapple				
Canned	3.5 oz	100	0	0
Fresh	1 slice	45	0	0
Potato salad	½ cup	150	9	54
Provolone	1 oz	90	7	70
Radishes	.5 oz	5	0	0
Red cabbage	¼ cup	5	0	0
Red onions	3 rings	5	0	0
Sesame sticks	1 oz	150	10	60
Shredded imitation				
cheese	1 oz	90	6	60
Soynuts	1 oz	120	7	52
Strawberries	2 oz	20	0	0
Sunflower seeds				
w/ raisins	1 oz	130	10	69
Swiss cheese	1 oz	105	8	67
Three-bean salad	½ cup	155	8	41
Tomatoes	1 oz	5	0	0
Turkey bits	2 oz	70	3	39
Turkey ham	¼ cup	50	2	36
Watermelon	2 pcs	20	0	0
Wine vinegar	1 tbsp	5	0	0

SALAD DRESSINGS

(Most ladles at salad bars hold 2 to 6 tablespoons of salad dressing.)

	AMOUNT	CALORIES	FAT-GRAMS	% FAT
Anchovy mayonnaise	2 tbsp	195	21	98
Bacon-tomato, reduced-calorie	2 tbsp	90	8	80
Bleu Lorraine dressing	2 tbsp	115	12	94
Blue cheese dressing	2 tbsp	149	16	97
Blue cheese French dressing	2 tbsp	185	20	98
Boiled dressing	2 tbsp	35	1	26
Buttermilk dressing	2 tbsp	50	3	55
Caesar dressing	2 tbsp	155	16	92
Caper dressing	2 tbsp	190	21	99
Celery seed dressing	2 tbsp	225	21	84
Chiffonade French dressing	2 tbsp	170	19	99
Chive French dressing	2 tbsp	185	20	98
Creamy cucumber, reduced-calorie	2 tbsp	100	10	90
Creamy garlic dressing	2 tbsp	150	16	97
Creamy Italian dressing	2 tbsp	165	18	99
Chutney dressing	2 tbsp	185	20	98
Cocktail sauce	2 tbsp	35	0	0
Cream cheese grenadine	2 tbsp	90	5	50
Cucumber dressing	2 tbsp	90	10	100
Curry dressing	2 tbsp	205	22	97
Dijon dressing	2 tbsp	150	17	100
Dill weed dressing	2 tbsp	85	9	96
French dressing	2 tbsp	185	20	98

	AMOUNT	CALORIES	FAT-GRAMS	% FAT
Fruit French dressing	2 tbsp	130	14	95
Garlic dressing	2 tbsp	155	17	99
Ginger dressing	2 tbsp	190	20	95
Ginger syrup	2 tbsp	90	0	0
Ginger vinaigrette	2 tbsp	170	18	94
Green Goddess dressing	2 tbsp	120	13	99
Guacamole dressing	2 tbsp	105	11	96
Honey fruit dressing	2 tbsp	50	3	55
Horseradish French dressing	2 tbsp	170	19	99
Hot bacon dressing	2 tbsp	235	15	57
Italian dressing	2 tbsp	145	14	86
Reduced-calorie	2 tbsp	50	4	72
Lemon ginger dressing	2 tbsp	85	7	75
Lemon syrup	2 tbsp	60	0	0
Lime syrup	2 tbsp	60	0	0
Louie sauce	2 tbsp	135	13	87
Mayonnaise	2 tbsp	200	22	98
Mustard mayonnaise	2 tbsp	155	17	97
Oil & vinegar dressing	2 tbsp	140	14	90
Oil-free dressing	2 tbsp	15	0	0
Orange & poppy seed vinaigrette	2 tbsp	180	18	91
Orange & poppy seed oil-free dressing	2 tbsp	35	0	0
Orange syrup	2 tbsp	75	0	0
Peanut butter dressing	2 tbsp	200	21	95
Pesto dressing	2 tbsp	140	14	90
Ranch-style dressing	2 tbsp	160	16	90
Remoulade dressing	2 tbsp	175	19	98

	AMOUNT	CALORIES	FAT-GRAMS	% FAT
Roquefort dressing	2 tbsp	120	12	91
Russian dressing	2 tbsp	135	14	93
Sesame dressing	2 tbsp	180	16	80
Sesame seed dressing	2 tbsp	225	21	84
Shogun dressing	2 tbsp	125	13	94
Sun-dried tomato vinaigrette	2 tbsp	75	3	36
Tartar sauce	2 tbsp	160	17	96
Thousand Island dressing	2 tbsp	165	17	93
Low-calorie	2 tbsp	35	2	50
Tomato-basil vinaigrette, low-calorie	2 tbsp	10	0	0
Tomato French dressing	2 tbsp	80	7	80
Tropical fruit dressing	2 tbsp	110	11	90
Victor dressing	2 tbsp	95	10	98
Vinaigrette	2 tbsp	170	18	94
Walnut vinaigrette dressing	2 tbsp	130	14	95
Yogurt dressing	2 tbsp	35	2	50
Zero dressing, low-calorie	2 tbsp	5	0	0

SANDWICHES

	AMOUNT	CALORIES	FAT GRAMS	% FAT
(Unless otherwise indicated, sandwiches are made with 2 slices of bread.)				
Bacon, lettuce & tomato sandwich (3 slices bacon) w/ mayo	1	420	21	45
Bacon, lettuce, tomato & avocado sandwich	1	490	30	55
Plain bagel	1	195	1	5
w/ 1 oz regular cream cheese	1	275	8	26
Bagel w/ cream cheese & smoked salmon or lox	1	425	21	44
Beef:				
BBQ roast beef on bun (w/ BBQ sauce)	1	250	8	29
Beef pocket sandwich (beef, lettuce & tomato in pita)	1	270	5	17
Coney Island sandwich (grilled ground beef & frankfurter, mayo & mustard on triple-decker bun)	1	635	46	65

	AMOUNT	CALORIES	FAT-GRAMS	% FAT
English pub beef (roast beef & horseradish dressing on Kaiser roll)	1	480	34	64
French dip	1	360	15	37
Hot roast beef sandwich w/ gravy	1	420	15	32
Italian beef (roast beef, peppers & onions on hoagie roll)	1	625	39	56
Italian meatball hero	1	535	25	42
Papa Joe's	1	280	11	35
Philly beef sandwich (roast beef, onions, mushrooms, melted cheese & dressing on French roll)	1	820	33	36
Roast beef sandwich w/o mayo	1	345	14	36
w/ cheese	1	400	18	40
Roast beef deluxe sandwich (feta cheese, lettuce, tomato, garlic, onion & olive oil in pita)	1	410	27	59
Sloppy joe	1	325	15	41
Steakball hero on French roll (3 meatballs)	1	470	22	43

	AMOUNT	CALORIES	FAT-GRAMS	% FAT
Bologna sandwich w/ mayo, lettuce & mustard	1	405	19	42
w/ cheese	1	425	28	59
Burgers:				
BBQ bacon burger (grilled beef, bacon, lettuce, tomato, cheese, mayo & BBQ sauce on bun)	1	700	46	59
BBQ burger (grilled beef & BBQ sauce on bun)	1	440	22	45
BBQ chicken burger (grilled chicken, lettuce, tomato, onion & BBQ sauce on bun)	1	320	6	17
BBQ chicken burger deluxe (grilled chicken, lettuce, tomato, onion, BBQ sauce, cheese & mayo on bun)	1	495	22	40
Border chicken burger (grilled chicken, cheese, green chilies, tomatoes & guacamole on hard roll)	1	965	68	63

	AMOUNT	CALORIES	FAT-GRAMS	% FAT
Canadian bacon cheese burger (grilled beef, cheese & Canadian bacon on bun)	1	570	34	53
Cheeseburger (w/o mayo or mayo-type dressing)	1	320	15	42
Double	1	545	28	46
Extra-large	1	610	33	49
Chicken cheeseburger (grilled chicken, cheese, lettuce, tomato & mayo on bun)	1	475	32	60
Chili guacamole burger (grilled beef, cheese, chili, tomatoes & guacamole on bun)	1	860	65	68
Deviled tuna cheeseburger (deviled tuna & cheese on bun)	1	405	24	53
French dip hamburger sandwich (grilled beef on French roll w/ au jus sauce)	1	410	20	44
w/ cheese	1	520	29	50
Grilled onion burger (grilled beef, lettuce, mayo & buttered grilled onions on bun)	1	565	38	60

SANDWICHES

	AMOUNT	CALORIES	FAT-GRAMS	% FAT
Guacamole burger (grilled beef, bacon, lettuce, tomato, mayo & guacamole on bun)	1	665	44	59
Hamburger (w/o mayo or mayo-type dressing)	1	275	12	39
Double	1	460	22	43
Extra-large	1	510	27	48
Mushroom burger (grilled beef & sautéed mushrooms on bun)	1	445	27	54
Patty melt (grilled beef & cheese on bread)	1	485	30	55
Peanut butter bacon burger (grilled beef, lettuce, tomato, mayo, bacon & peanut butter on bun)	1	765	53	62
Pizzaburger (grilled beef, mozzarella & pizza sauce on bun)	1	370	19	46
Refried bean burger (grilled beef, special sauce & refried beans on bun)	1	405	22	49

	AMOUNT	CALORIES	FAT-GRAMS	% FAT
Teriyaki burger (grilled ground beef, teriyaki sauce, cheese, tomato, lettuce, pineapple & mayo on bun)	1	635	41	58
Teriyaki chicken burger (chicken, teriyaki sauce, lettuce, tomato & onion on bun)	1	330	5	13
Turkey fillet burger deluxe (grilled turkey, bacon, tomato & cheese on bread)	1	445	25	50
Viennese schnitzelburger (grilled ground beef & fried egg on English muffin)	1	520	32	55
Cheese:				
French-fried cheese sandwich	1	590	33	50
Grilled cheese sandwich	1	360	23	57
w/ bacon		450	30	60
w/ chili		405	25	55
w/ ham		410	25	55
w/ olive		380	24	57
w/ tomato		370	23	56
Ham & cheese melt on hamburger bun	1	320	17	48
Hot provolone sandwich	1	380	18	43

	AMOUNT	CALORIES	FAT-GRAMS	% FAT
Chicken:				
Almond chicken salad sandwich	1	350	19	49
BBQ chicken burger (grilled chicken, lettuce, tomato, onion & BBQ sauce on bun)	1	320	6	17
Deluxe (grilled chicken, lettuce, tomato, onion, BBQ sauce, cheese & mayo on bun)	1	495	22	40
BBQ chicken burger deluxe (grilled chicken, lettuce, tomato, onion, BBQ sauce, cheese & mayo on bun)	1	495	22	40
Border chicken burger (grilled chicken, cheese, green chilies, tomatoes & guacamole on hard roll)	1	965	68	63
Chicken-avocado sandwich	1	480	30	56
Chicken breast sandwich (w/ mayo & lettuce)	1	320	12	34
Chicken Caesar wrap	1	630	31	44

	AMOUNT	CALORIES	FAT-GRAMS	% FAT
Chicken cheeseburger (grilled chicken, cheese, lettuce, tomato & mayo on bun)	1	475	32	60
Chicken club sandwich	1	545	26	43
Chicken fajita roll-up	1	705	36	43
Chicken mandarin salad sandwich (chicken salad & mandarin oranges on bread)	1	280	12	38
Chicken pocket sandwich (chicken, lettuce & tomato in pita)	1	255	3	10
Chicken salad sandwich	1	335	17	56
Chicken sandwich deluxe (chicken, lettuce, tomato, garlic, feta, onion & olive oil in pita)	1	395	25	57
Chicken submarine (chicken, cheese, lettuce, tomato, avocado & dressing on French roll)	1	480	24	45
Mediterranean chicken wrap	1	580	22	34
Southwestern chicken wrap	1	795	41	46
Teriyaki chicken burger (chicken, teriyaki sauce, lettuce, tomato & onion on bun)	1	330	5	13

	AMOUNT	CALORIES	FAT-GRAMS	% FAT
Coney Island sandwich (grilled ground beef & frankfurter, mayo & mustard on triple-decker bun)	1	635	46	65
Corn dog	1	330	20	55
Corned beef on rye sandwich	1	370	19	46
Deli-size (8 oz)	1	800	60	68
Crabmeat salad sandwich	1	270	11	37
Cube steak sandwich (w/ onions, Swiss cheese & dressing on French bread)	1	505	21	37
Denver sandwich	1	350	19	49
Egg:				
Egg & bacon sandwich (w/ mayo)	1	503	32	57
Egg & cheese pocket sandwich (w/ sautéed onions, mushrooms & peppers in pita)	½ pita	365	21	52
Egg salad pocket sandwich (w/ lettuce & tomato in pita)	1	255	8	28
Egg salad sandwich	1	255	9	32
Ham & egg salad sandwich	1	305	15	44

	AMOUNT	CALORIES	FAT GRAMS	% FAT
Mexican egg sandwich (poached egg, cheese, tomatoes & refried beans on ½ English muffin)	1	230	13	51
Tuna & egg salad sandwich	1	305	14	41
Welsh egg (egg salad, bacon, tomato & cheese on English muffin)	1	580	36	56
Fish sandwich (hot seafood, cheese & tomato on sourdough bread)	1	650	32	44
Frankfurters:				
BBQ frankfurter w/ bun	1	290	16	49
Coney Island sandwich (grilled ground beef & frankfurter, mayo & mustard on triple-decker bun)	1	635	46	65
Corn dog	1	330	20	55
Frankfurter & chili on bun	1	320	18	51
Frankfurter & sauerkraut on bun	1	280	16	52
Frankfurter, chili & cheese on bun	1	330	20	54

	AMOUNT	CALORIES	FAT-GRAMS	% FAT
Frankfurter deluxe (frankfurter, relish, ketchup & mustard on bun)	1	310	16	46
Frankfurter w/ bacon & cheese on bun	1	370	24	58
Franks & baked beans on bun	1	360	17	43
Sloppy franks on bun	1	430	28	59
Stuffed BBQ frankfurter on bun (bread dressing)	1	340	19	50
French dip	1	360	15	37
Gyro	1	505	23	41
Ham & cheese sandwich	1	390	24	55
Ham & egg salad sandwich	1	305	15	44
Ham & turkey salad sandwich	1	280	10	32
Ham salad sandwich	1	355	20	51
Ham sandwich				
w/ mayo	1	365	19	47
w/o mayo	1	285	16	51
Hot sandwiches:				
Hot chicken sandwich w/ gravy	1	345	10	26
Hot pork sandwich w/ gravy	1	420	18	38
Hot provolone sandwich	1	380	18	43

	AMOUNT	CALORIES	FAT-GRAMS	% FAT
Hot roast beef sandwich w/ gravy	1	420	15	32
Hot turkey sandwich w/ gravy	1	410	10	22
Pizza sandwich (French bread, cheese & pizza sauce)	1	375	23	55
Reuben sandwich	1	485	28	52
Turkey Divan on English muffin (w/ broccoli & Mornay sauce)	1	520	21	36
Italian hoagie (salami, ham, cheese, tomato, onion, peppers, lettuce & dressing on hoagie roll)	1	490	27	49
Italian sausage sandwich (w/ peppers, onion & olive on Italian roll)	1	620	44	64
Knockwurst sandwich (w/ mustard on French roll)	1	875	65	67
Liverwurst sandwich	1	305	14	41
Lobster salad sandwich	1	270	11	36
Mexican egg sandwich (poached egg, cheese, tomatoes & refried beans on ½ English muffin)	1	230	13	51

	AMOUNT	CALORIES	FAT-GRAMS	% FAT
Monte Cristo	1	405	22	49
Muffuletta sandwich	1	600	31	46
New York steak sandwich (grilled lean New York steak on French roll)	1	340	13	34
Oyster sandwich, fried	1	710	23	29
Peanut butter sandwiches:				
Peanut butter & jelly sandwich	1	360	19	48
Peanut butter bacon burger (grilled ground beef, lettuce, tomato, mayo, bacon & peanut butter on bun)	1	765	53	62
Peanut butter sandwich	1	340	19	50
Sesame Street club sandwich (peanut butter, bacon, lettuce & tomato)	1	570	33	52
Philly beef sandwich (roast beef, onions, mushrooms, melted cheese & dressing on French roll)	1	820	33	36

	AMOUNT	CALORIES	FAT-GRAMS	% FAT
Pocket sandwiches (in pita bread):				
Beef pocket sandwich (beef, lettuce & tomato)	1	270	5	17
Beef pocket sandwich deluxe (roast beef, feta, lettuce, tomato, garlic, onion & olive oil)	1	410	27	59
Chicken pocket sandwich (chicken, lettuce & tomato)	1	255	3	10
Chicken pocket sandwich deluxe (chicken, lettuce, tomato, garlic, feta, onion & olive oil)	1	395	25	57
Egg & cheese pocket sandwich (w/ sautéed onions, mushrooms & peppers)	½ pita	365	21	52
Egg salad pocket sandwich (w/ lettuce & tomato)	1	255	8	28
Veggie pocket sandwich (sprouts, onion, olives, tomatoes, mayo, lettuce & mushrooms)	1	340	18	47

SANDWICHES

	AMOUNT	CALORIES	FAT-GRAMS	% FAT
w/ avocado		495	32	58
w/ avocado & cheese		610	41	61
w/ cheese		455	27	53
Polish sausage sandwich (w/ Swiss cheese & sauerkraut on bun)	1	565	41	65
Pork:				
BBQ pork (w/ BBQ sauce on French roll)	1	280	7	22
Hot pork sandwich w/ gravy	1	420	18	38
Salami sandwich	1	480	34	64
Salmon salad sandwich	1	275	12	39
Seafood salad sandwich	1	280	11	36
Sesame Street club sandwich (peanut butter, bacon, lettuce & tomato)	1	570	33	52
Shrimp club sandwich	1	515	26	45
Shrimp croissant sandwich	1	365	24	59
Shrimp salad sandwich	1	290	14	43
Curried	1	295	14	43
Stromboli boat (spicy ground beef, & mozzarella on Kaiser roll)	1	330	17	46

	AMOUNT	CALORIES	FAT-GRAMS	% FAT
Submarine sandwich (salami, pepperoni, summer sausage, provolone, Swiss cheese, mozzarella, mayo, mustard, lettuce & tomato on French roll)	1	540	29	48
Thai vegetable roll	1	445	8	16
Tuna:				
Deviled tuna cheeseburger (deviled tuna & cheese on bun)	1	405	24	53
Grilled tuna w/ cheese on rye	1	490	26	48
Southwestern tuna wrap	1	950	64	61
Tuna & egg salad sandwich	1	305	14	41
Tuna finger sandwiches	2 slices	290	14	43
Tuna fish salad sandwich	1	310	14	40
Tuna patty sandwich (patty, cheese, lettuce, tomato & tartar sauce)	1	505	32	57
Tuna sandwich Italian-style (tuna salad, peppers, onion, pizza sauce & mozzarella on torpedo roll)	1	485	27	50

	AMOUNT	CALORIES	FAT-GRAMS	% FAT
Turkey:				
Ham & turkey salad sandwich	1	280	10	32
Hot turkey sandwich w/ gravy	1	340	10	26
Oriental turkey salad sandwich (diced turkey, celery, grapes, water chestnuts & mayo)	1	285	12	38
Turkey & cream cheese sandwich w/ cranberry chutney	1	470	28	54
Turkey breast sandwich w/ mayo	1	420	18	39
w/o mayo	1	380	7	20
Turkey Divan on English muffin (w/ broccoli & Mornay sauce)	1	520	21	36
Turkey fillet burger deluxe (grilled turkey, bacon, tomato & cheese on bread)	1	445	25	50
Turkey sandwich deluxe (w/ bacon, cheese, lettuce, tomato & dressing on 1 slice bread)	1	475	24	45

	AMOUNT	CALORIES	FAT-GRAMS	% FAT
Veggie fajita wrap	1	460	23	45
Veggie-filled croissant sandwich w/ cheese	1	475	30	57
Veggie pocket sandwich (sprouts, onion, olives, tomatoes, mayo, lettuce & mushrooms in pita)	1	340	18	47
w/ avocado		495	32	58
w/ avocado & cheese		610	41	61
w/ cheese		455	27	53
Veggie sandwich (sprouts, onion, olives, tomatoes, lettuce, mayo & mushrooms)	1	340	19	50
w/ avocado		494	33	60
w/ avocado & cheese		610	42	62
w/ cheese		455	28	55
Viennese schnitzelburger (ground beef & fried egg on English muffin)	1	520	32	55
Welsh egg (egg salad, bacon, tomato & cheese on English muffin)	1	580	36	56

SAUCES, SPREADS & TABLE FATS

	AMOUNT	CALORIES	FAT-GRAMS	% FAT
A.1. Steak sauce	1 tbsp	15	0	0
Aioli sauce	2 tbsp	195	21	98
Au jus	2 tbsp	55	6	96
Bacon sauce	¼ cup	185	14	69
Barbecue sauce	2 tbsp	15	0	0
Béarnaise sauce	¼ cup	220	22	89
Béchamel sauce	¼ cup	90	7	68
Bordelaise sauce	¼ cup	45	3	57
Brown sauce	¼ cup	20	0	0
Butter	1 pat	35	4	100
	1 tsp	35	4	100
Whipped	1 tsp	25	3	100
Butter oil	1 tbsp	115	13	100
Butter sauce	2 tbsp	205	23	100
Caper sauce	¼ cup	135	11	74
Cardinal sauce	¼ cup	95	7	66
Champagne sauce	¼ cup	115	40	79
Chateaubriand sauce	¼ cup	65	6	84
Cheese sauce	¼ cup	105	8	68
Cherry sauce	2 tbsp	25	0	0
Cocktail sauce	2 tbsp	35	0	0

	AMOUNT	CALORIES	FAT-GRAMS	% FAT
Coffee lighteners, nondairy				
Liquid	1 tbsp	20	2	90
Powdered	1 tsp	10	1	90
Cranberry sauce	¼ cup	90	0	0
Cream:				
Light				
Coffee or table	1 tbsp	30	3	90
Whipping				
Unwhipped	1 tbsp	45	5	94
Whipped	2 tbsp	45	5	94
Half-and-half	1 tbsp	20	2	78
Heavy, whipping				
Unwhipped	1 tbsp	50	6	97
Whipped	2 tbsp	50	6	97
Cream sauce	¼ cup	80	6	66
Cucumber sauce	¼ cup	85	8	83
Cumberland sauce	2 tbsp	70	0	0
Daikon				
(Chinese horseradish)	⅓ cup	15	0	0
Dijonnaise sauce	¼ cup	65	5	69
Duxelles sauce	¼ cup	80	6	69
Enchilada sauce	¼ cup	25	1	37
Gravy	¼ cup	80	6	67
Guacamole sauce	2 tbsp	40	4	88
Hollandaise sauce	2 tbsp	185	20	97
Horseradish sauce	¼ cup	65	4	56
Horseradish sour cream	2 tbsp	100	11	99
Ketchup	1 tbsp	20	0	0
Kirsch sauce	¼ cup	140	9	58
Lemon butter	2 tbsp	55	5	83

SAUCES/SPREADS/TABLE FATS

	AMOUNT	CALORIES	FAT-GRAMS	% FAT
Lyonnaise sauce	¼ cup	45	2	38
Madeira sauce	¼ cup	30	1	28
Margarine				
Hard	1 pat	35	4	100
	1 tsp	35	4	100
Soft	1 tsp	35	4	100
Diet	1 pat	20	2	90
	1 tsp	20	2	90
Mayonnaise	1 tbsp	100	11	99
Light	1 tbsp	50	5	90
Nonfat	1 tbsp	10	0	0
Meunière sauce	¼ cup	200	22	99
Milanaise sauce	¼ cup	65	4	54
Mock Hollandaise sauce	2 tbsp	95	9	85
Mornay sauce	¼ cup	100	7	62
Mousseline sauce	¼ cup	200	20	90
Mushroom sauce	¼ cup	90	6	60
Mustard	1 tbsp	5	0	0
Mustard sauce	¼ cup	95	6	58
Hot	1 tbsp	25	0	0
Oriental	1 tbsp	35	2	51
Newburg sauce	¼ cup	110	9	73
Oils:				
Corn	1 tsp	40	5	100
Cottonseed	1 tsp	40	5	100
Olive	1 tsp	40	5	100
Peanut	1 tsp	40	5	100
Rapeseed (canola)	1 tsp	40	5	100
Safflower	1 tsp	40	5	100
Sunflower	1 tsp	40	5	100

	AMOUNT	CALORIES	FAT GRAMS	% FAT
Orange sauce	¼ cup	105	0	0
Oyster sauce	¼ cup	110	7	58
Pesto	1 tbsp	155	15	86
Piquante sauce	¼ cup	25	0	0
Sabayon sauce	¼ cup	55	3	49
Sour cream				
Regular	1 tbsp	25	3	90
Low-fat	1 tbsp	20	1	45
Nonfat	1 tbsp	20	0	0
Sweet pickle relish	1 tbsp	20	0	0
Sweet-and-sour sauce	1 tbsp	30	0	0
Tabasco	¼ cup	0	0	0
Tartar sauce	1 tbsp	70	8	100
Teriyaki sauce	1 tbsp	30	0	0
Velouté sauce	¼ cup	65	5	67
Worcestershire sauce	1 tbsp	60	0	0

SEAFOOD

	AMOUNT	CALORIES	FAT-GRAMS	% FAT
Abalone, fried	7 oz	210	2	8
Baked fish	5 oz	245	11	40
Bass:				
Bass fillet w/ sorrel				
& cream sauce	7 oz	390	21	48
Bass fillet, fried	7 oz	400	18	41
Sea bass in champagne				
& butter sauce	8 oz	480	27	51
Sea bass w/ shrimp				
stuffing	8 oz	415	12	24
Bluefish:				
Baked	8 pz	280	10	32
Cheese casserole	10 oz	455	22	43
Blackened fish	6.5 oz	390	20	46
Bouillabaisse	10 oz	235	9	35
Broiled fish	5 oz	245	11	40
Catfish				
Blackened	6.5 oz	390	20	46
Breaded & fried	6 oz	400	24	54
Cioppino	12 oz	440	17	35
Clams:				
Breaded & fried clams	20 sm	380	21	50
Cherrystone clams	9 lg	135	2	13

	AMOUNT	CALORIES	FAT-GRAMS	% FAT
Clams & chips				
(4 oz clams,				
4 oz fries)	1 serving	650	28	39
Clam fritters	3 oz	170	9	48
Deviled clam patties	4 oz	320	14	39
Fried clams	6 oz	380	20	47
Steamed clams				
(1 1b in shells)	20 sm	135	2	13
w/ fresh tomatoes,				
basil & garlic		265	8	28
w/ olive oil & lemon		335	21	56
Cod:				
Codfish cakes				
(2 oz each)	2	340	14	37
Dill smoked cod	5 oz	150	3	18
Fish & chips				
(4 oz cod, 4 oz fries)	1 serving	575	27	42
Scrod, breaded				
& fried	6 oz	400	24	54
Crab:				
Alaskan crab legs				
(6 oz)	1 leg	145	1	6
Crab in black bean				
sauce	½ crab	330	24	66
Crab cakes (2 oz each)	2	240	15	56
Crab gumbo	8 oz	105	4	34
Crab Imperial	8 oz	450	32	64
Crabmeat au gratin	6 oz	285	16	50
Crabmeat & macaroni				
Newburg	8 oz	305	14	41

	AMOUNT	CALORIES	FAT-GRAMS	% FAT
Crab Mornay (crab, mushrooms, cheese sauce, toast)	main dish	500	34	61
Crabmeat salad sandwich	1	270	11	37
Crab tostada (crab, beans, cheese, olives, avocado, sour cream)	1	920	47	46
Deviled crab	5 oz	225	13	52
Dungeness crab, cracked	2 lb crab	230	4	16
Dungeness crab in cream sauce (crab, asparagus, avocado, jack cheese)	1 crab	715	45	56
Fried soft-shell blue crab	1 lg	320	23	65
Herb-seasoned cracked crab	½ crab	240	14	53
Imitation crab	3 oz	85	1	10
King crabmeat soufflé (4" × 6")	1 servng	310	16	47
Crawfish étouffée (crawfish, rice)	8 oz	390	17	39
Deep-fat fried fish	4 oz	440	19	39
Fillets Florentine	4 oz	230	10	39
Fillets piccata	4 oz	300	22	66

	AMOUNT	CALORIES	FAT-GRAMS	% FAT
Fillets w/ beer-cheese sauce	6 oz	600	42	63
Fish & chips (4 oz fish, 4 oz fries)	1 serving	575	27	42
Fish chowder	6 oz	100	5	44
Fish sandwich (hot seafood, cheese & tomato on sourdough bread)	1	650	32	44
Fish taco (fish, lettuce, sour cream)	1	265	15	51
Fisherman's platter (5 pcs fish, 2.5 oz fries)	1 serving	730	40	49
Flounder				
Fried	7 oz	400	16	36
Stuffed w/ lobster	8 oz	545	33	54
Haddock:				
Baked haddock in Newburg sauce	5 oz	400	21	47
Fried	7 oz	320	12	34
Haddock fillet platter (w/ potatoes, tomatoes, mushrooms)	5 oz	875	54	56
Halibut:				
Broiled halibut	5 oz	245	11	40
Halibut w/ cream sherry sauce	5 oz	315	17	49

	AMOUNT	CALORIES	FAT-GRAMS	% FAT
Halibut fillet				
Amandine	4 oz	255	17	60
à l'orange (5 oz fillet, 2 oz sauce)	1 serving	320	12	34
Halibut steak, baked	5 oz	245	11	40
Lobster-stuffed halibut fillets w/ Newburg sauce	8 oz	500	30	54
Pan-fried halibut (breaded)	5 oz	395	17	39
Poached halibut	5 oz	180	4	20
Herring				
Kippered	1 med pc	85	5	53
Pickled	½ oz	40	3	67
Lobster:				
Boiled or steamed lobster	1.25 lb	220	1	8
Broiled lobster tail beurre	8 oz	335	16	45
Crumb-topped lobster tails	1 tail	170	7	37
Lobster w/ crab stuffing & creamy cheese sauce	1 lobster	695	49	63
Lobster Newburg (w/o rice)	6 oz	70	3	37
w/ 1 popover		320	17	48
Lobster-stuffed halibut fillets w/ Newburg sauce	8 oz	500	30	54

	AMOUNT	CALORIES	FAT-GRAMS	% FAT
Lobster thermidor	5 oz ramekin	190	10	47
Steamed lobster tail	6 oz	175	1	5
Mixed seafood grill	4 oz	280	9	29
Monkfish, baked	7 oz	150	2	12
Mussels:				
Mussels & clams, steamed in wine & garlic (½ lb in shells)	1 serving	205	5	23
Mussels marinara	½ lb	210	8	34
Steamed mussels in olive oil, garlic & tomatoes	1 doz	330	12	33
Orange roughy, grilled	5 oz	210	10	43
Pan-fried fish	5 oz	395	17	39
Poached fish	5 oz	180	4	20
Portuguese fish stew	12 oz	475	21	40
Oysters:				
Fried oysters	3 lg	200	11	49
Oysters au gratin	8 oz	295	18	55
Oysters Rockefeller	3	80	5	58
Oysters topped w/ bacon, crab & Newburg sauce	6	280	14	45
Raw oysters	6 med	70	2	26
Scalloped oysters	8 oz	400	20	45
Redfish:				
Blackened redfish	3.5 oz	195	11	51
Cajun redfish	3.5 oz	195	11	51

SEAFOOD

	AMOUNT	CALORIES	FAT-GRAMS	% FAT
Red mullet Triestina (fish, wine, lemon juice, capers, fried bread)	8 oz	475	17	32
Red snapper Liguria (fish, tomato, wine sauce, anchovies)	8 oz	405	12	26
Rockfish amandine	8 oz	565	35	56
Salmon:				
Alder-smoked salmon	6 oz	265	16	54
BBQ salmon	6 oz	265	16	54
Hickory-smoked salmon	6 oz	265	16	54
Poached salmon	8 oz	265	8	27
Salmon cake	3.5 oz	240	15	56
Salmon croquettes	4 oz	370	19	46
Salmon coulibiac (fish, rice, puff pastry)	1 serving	1,640	108	59
Salmon in crust	12 oz	915	48	47
Salmon loaf	5 oz	205	9	40
Salmon, noodles & mushroom casserole	12 oz	595	32	48
Salmon quiche (crustless)	⅙ of 9" quiche	280	17	55
Salmon salad sandwich	1	275	12	39
Salmon shortcake (creamed salmon, 1 biscuit)	1 serving	495	28	51

	AMOUNT	CALORIES	FAT-GRAMS	% FAT
Salmon teriyaki	6 oz	260	6	21
Salmon topped				
w/ guacamole sauce				
& sour cream	6 oz	635	46	65
Scalloped salmon	5 oz	205	9	40
Smoked salmon	3 oz	100	4	36
w/ cream cheese				
& bagel	1 serving	425	21	44
Stuffed salmon				
(garden vegetable				
stuffing)	6 oz	330	20	54
Scallops:				
Broiled scallops				
w/ ginger soy sauce	5 oz	155	6	35
Coquilles St. Jacques	5 oz			
	ramekin	220	10	41
Fried scallops	5 oz	285	11	36
Imitation scallops	3 oz	85	0	0
Scallops & prawns				
w/ risotto	9 oz	445	5	10
Scallops Dijonnaise	4 oz	215	11	46
Scallops en brochette	1			
	brochette	290	7	22
Scallops in garlic butter	5 oz	270	16	53
Scallops w/ fettuccine				
in cream sauce	10 oz	1,000	61	55
Scrod, breaded & fried	6 oz	400	24	54
Seafood à la meunière				
(seafood fillet,				
white sauce)	5 oz	445	33	67

	AMOUNT	CALORIES	FAT-GRAMS	% FAT
Seafood, breaded & fried	6 oz	400	24	54
Seafood brochette	1	170	3	16
Seafood cakes	4 oz	340	14	37
Seafood fillets amandine	4 oz	255	17	60
Seafood in cream sauce	5 oz	315	17	49
Seafood, meat & vegetable chow mein				
w/ pan-fried noodles	main dish	680	36	48
w/ soft noodles	12 oz	565	30	48
Seafood medley (shrimp, scallops, prawns, halibut, Cajun sauce)	4 oz	360	14	35
Seafood pot pie	1	555	31	50
Seafood risotto	9 oz	445	5	10
Seafood salad sandwich	1	280	11	36
Shark teriyaki	4 oz	140	5	32
Shellfish:				
Imitation shellfish (surimi)	3 oz	85	1	11
Shellfish medley w/ aioli sauce (clams, mussels, crab, shrimp)	8 oz	355	6	15
Shrimp:				
Bahia shrimp stir-fry	8 oz	305	19	56
Baked stuffed prawns	6 prawns	340	19	50
BBQ shrimp	6 oz	255	2	70
Beer-batter shrimp	6 oz	410	26	57

	Amount	Calories	Fat-Grams	% Fat
Boiled shrimp	5 oz	155	2	12
Butterflied shrimp teriyaki	6 oz	255	1	35
Cajun shrimp	6 oz	255	2	70
Cajun shrimp kabobs	1 kabob	221	8	32
Chinese fried shrimp	6 oz	535	28	47
French-fried breaded shrimp	6 oz	410	26	57
Grilled prawns w/ tomato & basil	3 prawns	270	16	54
Hong Kong shrimp (⅔ cup shrimp, vegetables, 1 cup rice)	1 serving	640	8	11
Imitation shrimp	3 oz	85	1	10
Peel & eat shrimp	5 oz	155	2	12
Phoenix-tail shrimp	4 oz	305	12	36
per 1 tbsp dipping sauce	add	29	0	0
Prawns & scallops in lemon cream sauce	5 oz	375	18	43
Princess prawns (fried prawns, cashews, hot sauce)	8 oz	505	25	44
Shrimp & noodles au gratin	6 oz	265	12	41
Shrimp Calypso (shrimp, butter, brandy, tomato sauce)	8 oz	415	26	56

	AMOUNT	CALORIES	FAT-GRAMS	% FAT
Shrimp chimichanga (shrimp, cheese, tortilla, sour cream)	1 serving	595	35	53
Shrimp chow mein (w/o noodles)	1 cup	220	10	41
Shrimp club sandwich	1	515	26	45
Shrimp croissant sandwich	1	365	24	59
Shrimp Creole	8 oz	300	9	27
Shrimp curry (w/o rice)	6 oz	235	14	53
Shrimp De Jonghe	6 shrimp	340	19	50
Shrimp enchilada (w/o topping)	1	370	21	51
Shrimp fried rice	8 oz	320	10	28
Shrimp gumbo	8 oz	105	4	34
Shrimp jambalaya (shrimp, rice, ham, peppers, tomato sauce)	8 oz	290	8	25
Shrimp rice casserole (2 oz shirmp, 1½ cups rice, sauce)	1 serving	360	13	33
Shrimp salad sandwich	1	290	14	43
Shrimp scampi	3 oz	230	16	63
w/ saffron rice	6 shrimp	825	49	53
Shrimp Siciliano (shrimp, tomato, red wine sauce)	8 oz	415	26	56

	AMOUNT	CALORIES	FAT-GRAMS	% FAT
Shrimp tostada (beans, cheese, avocado, sour cream)	1	940	47	45
Shrimp w/ bean curd & vegetable	12 oz	520	21	36
Shrimp w/ garlic butter	4 oz	320	27	76
Shrimp w/ lobster sauce	4 oz	345	16	42
Shrimp w/ peppers	4 oz	165	5	27
Sizzling rice shrimp	8 oz	460	19	37
Stir-fried shrimp				
w/ snow peas	8 oz	245	12	44
w/ vegetables	8 oz	245	18	66
Sweet-and-sour shrimp	6 oz	235	12	46
Sizzling sweet-and-sour seafood	8 oz	460	19	37
Sole:				
Broccoli-stuffed sole	4 oz	460	25	49
Fillet of sole Florentine	6 oz	365	15	37
Sole à la Bonne Femme (sole, mushrooms, cream sauce)	6 oz	415	18	39
Sole in sweet-and-sour sauce	4 oz	460	29	57
Sole le Marmère (breaded & fried)	6 oz	605	37	55
Sole w/ shrimp, crab & mushroom stuffing	5 oz	340	15	39

	AMOUNT	CALORIES	FAT-GRAMS	% FAT
Squid:				
Calamari Milanese (squid, egg batter, white wine, capers, lemon)	3 oz	190	11	52
Calamari w/ linguine (squid, linguine, tomato sauce, clams)	1.5 cup	410	6	13
Fried squid	5 oz	248	11	40
Squid & snow peas stir-fry w/ noodles	main dish	475	19	36
Squid & vegetable stir fry	main dish	215	11	46
Stir-fried calamari	5 oz	248	11	40
Stuffed squid	8 oz	285	10	31
Sturgeon, smoked	3 oz	145	4	24
Sushi or sashimi	3.5 oz	145	5	31
Sweet-and-sour seafood kabob	1	205	5	22
Swordfish:				
Broiled swordfish steak w/ olive oil,	8 oz	410	14	30
garlic, lemon	8 oz	600	45	68
Grilled swordfish steak puttanesca	5 oz	410	32	70
Marinated grilled swordfish steak	4 oz	180	10	50
Swordfish kabob	1	150	7	42

	AMOUNT	CALORIES	FAT-GRAMS	% FAT
Tempura fish fillet	1	440	21	51
Trout:				
Grilled rainbow trout	4 oz	245	12	44
Stuffed trout				
(⅓ cup bread stuffing)	1 trout	595	40	60
w/ Swiss chard		395	30	68
Trout sauté amandine	4	235	12	46
Tuna:				
Creamed tuna w/ peas	6 oz	240	11	41
Grilled tuna w/ fresh				
tomato & basil				
sauce		345	21	55
Grilled tuna sandwich				
w/ cheese on rye	1	490	26	48
Mandarin tuna				
(tuna, rice, noodles,				
vegetables, sauce)	8 oz	520	17	29
Scalloped tuna	5 oz	205	9	40
Southwestern tuna				
wrap	1	950	64	61
Tuna à la king	6 oz	275	11	36
Tuna & celery on				
crackers	3 oz	305	15	44
Tuna & egg salad				
sandwich	1	305	14	41
Tuna fish turnover	1	375	23	55
Tuna fish salad				
sandwich	1	310	14	40
Tuna Florentine	8 oz	520	42	72
Tuna loaf	5 oz	355	24	61

	AMOUNT	CALORIES	FAT-GRAMS	% FAT
Tuna noodle casserole	8 oz	300	12	36
Tuna patty sandwich (patty, cheese, lettuce, tomato & tartar sauce)	1	505	32	57
Tuna rarebit	8 oz	315	17	48
Tuna rice casserole	8 oz	210	8	34
Tuna sandwich Italian-style (tuna salad, peppers, onion, pizza sauce & mozzarella on torpedo roll)	1	485	27	50
Tuna tetrazzini	8 oz	505	18	32
Whitefish:				
Broiled whitefish amandine	8 oz	655	49	67
Mediterranean whitefish (fish, olive oil, lemon, onions)	8 oz	260	8	27
Smoked whitefish	3 oz	90	1	10
Whitefish stuffed w/ wild rice	8 oz	428	17	36

SOUPS

	AMOUNT	CALORIES	FAT-GRAMS	% FAT
Avgolemono soup	8 oz	185	5	24
Barley soups:				
Barley & mushroom soup	8 oz	180	7	35
Cream of barley w/ prosciutto	10 oz	340	20	53
Scotch barley	6 oz	75	2	24
Bean soup	8 oz	185	5	24
Bisques:				
Clam	6 oz	240	16	59
Oyster	6 oz	330	15	57
Shrimp	6 oz	175	13	67
Black bean soup	8 oz	180	5	23
Beef broth	8 oz	20	1	45
Beef Calcutta (beef stock, beef, vegetables, rice curry, apple)	6 oz	105	5	43
Beef consommé	8 oz	30	0	0
Beef noodle soup	6 oz	5	1	16
Beef rice soup	6 oz	55	1	16
Beef soup w/ farina dumpling	8 oz	65	3	42

	AMOUNT	CALORIES	FAT-GRAMS	% FAT
Blueberry soup				
w/ cream	8 oz	125	6	43
Borscht				
(w/ 2 tbsp sour cream)	8 oz	90	6	59
Polish-style				
(w/ duck & sausage)	8 oz	110	8	67
Bouillabaisse	12 oz	235	9	35
Cabbage soups:				
Old-fashioned cabbage				
soup	8 oz	165	10	54
Sauerkraut soup	8 oz	175	14	72
Viennese cabbage soup				
(w/ Polish sausage)	8 oz	240	20	75
Cajun Creole soup	6 oz	75	1	12
Cheddar cheese soup	6 oz	170	11	57
Chicken Acapulco				
(chicken broth,				
chicken, avocado,				
tortilla, cheese)	8 oz	280	13	41
Chicken broth	8 oz	35	1	26
Chicken consommé	8 oz	30	0	0
Chicken Calcutta				
(chicken, stock,				
vegetables, rice,				
curry, apple)	6 oz	105	5	43
Chicken corn chowder	8 oz	115	6	46
Chicken giblets w/ rice	6 oz	80	4	45
Chicken gumbo	8 oz	125	5	36
Chicken mulligatawny	6 oz	110	6	48
Chicken noodle soup	6 oz	80	2	22

	AMOUNT	CALORIES	FAT-GRAMS	% FAT
Chicken vegetable soup	6 oz	65	1	14
Chili	6 oz	150	4	24
Clam bisque	6 oz	240	16	59
Chowders:				
Chicken corn chowder	8 oz	115	6	46
Clam chowder				
Boston	6 oz	140	7	46
Manhattan	6 oz	130	6	41
New England	6 oz	225	12	48
Corn chowder	6 oz	235	11	42
Crab chowder	6 oz	110	5	40
Fish chowder	6 oz	100	5	44
Potato chowder	6 oz	150	7	41
Turkey chowder	8 oz	125	3	22
Vegetable chowder	6 oz	85	5	52
Cioppino	12 oz	440	17	35
Cock-a-leekie	8 oz	185	4	20
Continental bean				
w/ bacon strip	6 oz	330	22	60
Corn chowder	6 oz	235	11	42
Country vegetable soup	6 oz	60	0	0
Crab chowder	6 oz	110	5	40
Crab gumbo	8 oz	105	4	34
Cream soups:				
Cream of almond	6 oz	205	16	70
Cream of asparagus	8 oz	170	10	53
Cream of broccoli	8 oz	155	11	64
Cream of carrot	6 oz	265	17	57
Cream of celery	6 oz	235	16	61
Cream of chicken	6 oz	245	15	55

SOUPS

	AMOUNT	CALORIES	FAT-GRAMS	% FAT
Cream of mushroom	6 oz	280	19	61
Cream of oyster	8 oz	160	7	40
Cream of spinach	6 oz	215	14	59
Cream of tomato	6 oz	170	9	48
Cream of vegetable	6 oz	195	11	51
Duchess	6 oz	225	14	56
Duchess cream of tomato	6 oz	155	8	46
Duck soup Parisienne	8 oz	20	1	41
Dutch vegetable soup	6 oz	170	10	53
Egg drop soup	6 oz	70	4	51
Fish chowder	6 oz	100	5	44
French onion soup	8 oz	385	25	58
Gazpacho	1 cup	45	0	0
Genovese fish soup	8 oz	480	20	37
Goulash soup	8 oz	215	10	42
Guacamole soup	4 oz	115	9	70
Gumbos:				
Chicken	8 oz	125	5	36
Crab	8 oz	105	4	34
Shrimp	8 oz	105	4	34
Turkey	8 oz	95	4	38
Hot-and-sour soup	8 oz	75	2	24
Jellied chicken consommé	6 oz	40	1	21
Jellied tomato madrilene	6 oz	40	0	0
Lamb broth Anglaise	8 oz	115	5	39
Lentil soup	6 oz	300	19	57
Lima bean & bacon soup	6 oz	280	21	68

	AMOUNT	CALORIES	FAT-GRAMS	% FAT
Manhattan clam chowder	6 oz	130	6	41
Minestrone Italiano	6 oz	155	4	23
Minestrone w/ pesto	8 oz	220	7	29
Miso soup	8 oz	50	1	18
Navy bean soup	8 oz	185	5	24
New England clam chowder	6 oz	225	12	48
Old-fashioned cabbage soup	8 oz	165	10	54
Olla podrida (black-eyed peas, rice, chorizo, sausage, chicken, ham, garbanzo beans, chicken stock)	8 oz	175	14	72
Onion soup	6 oz	95	5	47
Oxtail soup	8 oz	170	8	42
Oxtail soup à l'Anglaise	8 oz	125	5	35
Oyster bisque	6 oz	240	15	57
Oyster stew	8 oz	220	12	49
Pea soup:				
Green pea	8 oz	133	2	13
Split	8 oz	200	3	13
Philadelphia pepper pot	6 oz	125	6	43
Polish lentil soup	6 oz	300	19	57
Potato & leek soup	6 oz	195	12	55
Potato chowder	6 oz	150	7	41
Pot-au-feu	8 oz	135	5	33
Puree Mongol	6 oz	280	18	58

SOUPS

	AMOUNT	CALORIES	FAT-GRAMS	% FAT
Raspberry crème (cold)	6 oz	100	1	9
Rice soup Florentine	8 oz	130	6	41
Sauerkraut soup	8 oz	175	14	72
Sausage & vegetable soup	8 oz	365	21	52
Shark fin soup	8 oz	195	5	23
Shrimp bisque	6 oz	175	13	67
Shrimp gumbo	8 oz	105	4	34
Sizzling rice soup	8 oz	170	5	26
Sopa Royale (chicken stock, sherry, pimento, chicken, eggs, ham)	8 oz	100	4	36
Snapper soup	6 oz	230	9	35
Split-pea soup	6 oz	350	18	46
Stracciatella (egg & cheese soup)	8 oz	65	3	42
Tomato bouillon w/ rice	8 oz	65	1	14
Tomato rice soup	6 oz	135	5	33
Tortellini chicken soup	10 oz	310	10	29
Tortellini vegetable soup	10 oz	300	89	24
Turkey chowder	8 oz	125	3	22
Turkey Creole soup	8 oz	85	5	53
Turkey gumbo	8 oz	95	4	38
Turkish cucumber Iman	8 oz	130	8	56
Turtle soup (clear)	8 oz	60	0	0
Tuscan tomato soup (basil, tomato soup, toasted bread, olive oil)	8 oz	295	14	43

	AMOUNT	CALORIES	FAT-GRAMS	% FAT
Vegetable chowder	6 oz	85	5	52
Vegetable, pasta & bean soup	10 oz	310	8	23
Viennese cabbage soup (w/ Polish sausage)	8 oz	240	20	75
Wonton soup	8 oz	195	11	51
Zupp'alla Roma (escarole & cheese soup)	8 oz	115	7	54

VEGETABLES

	AMOUNT	CALORIES	FAT-GRAMS	% FAT

(It may be assumed that vegetables served in most restaurants are cooked and/or served with a dollop or pat of butter.)

Artichokes:

	AMOUNT	CALORIES	FAT-GRAMS	% FAT
Artichoke hearts sauté	½ cup	100	8	72
Artichokes au gratin	½ cup	150	7	42
Artichoke w/ butter sauce	1	265	23	78
Herbed Jerusalem artichokes	½ cup	130	12	83
Whole artichoke, steamed	1	55	0	0
Artichoke hearts, steamed	½ cup	40	0	0
Asparagus:				
Boiled/steamed	4 spears	15	0	0
Buttered	4 spears	35	2	53
Asparagus casserole	6 oz	165	10	54
Asparagus Dijon	½ cup	120	10	76
Asparagus-tomato stir-fry	½ cup	75	4	49
Lemon-buttered asparagus	½ cup	40	2	45

	AMOUNT	CALORIES	FAT-GRAMS	% FAT
Bavarian cabbage	½ cup	115	7	55
Beans & legumes:				
Baked beans	1 cup	240	2	7
Bean stew (kidney beans, tomatoes, onions, peppers)	½ cup	105	3	25
Black beans	1 cup	235	2	8
Black beans & rice (no fat added)	1 cup	315	1	3
Black-eyed peas	½ cup	140	2	13
(no fat added)	½ cup	100	1	4
Boston baked beans	1 cup	345	10	26
Broad beans, cooked	1 cup	190	1	5
Bruna boner (Swedish beans)	½ cup	210	2	8
Chili:				
Beef chili verde	1 cup	270	15	50
Chili con carne	1 cup	350	21	54
Chili w/ macaroni	1 cup	255	6	21
Beef	10 oz	340	17	45
Lamb	6 oz	260	13	45
Mexican pork chili	1 cup	590	41	63
San Antone chili	1 cup	590	41	63
Taos chili verde	1 cup	270	15	50
Fava beans, cooked	1 cup	180	1	5
French beans, steamed	1 cup	230	1	4
Gaucho beans (pinto beans, ground beef, bacon, tomatoes, seasoning)	1 cup	315	12	34

	AMOUNT	CALORIES	FAT-GRAMS	% FAT
Green beans	½ cup	20	0	0
& mushrooms				
(no fat added)	½ cup	25	0	0
& water chestnuts	½ cup	65	4	57
Amandine	½ cup	85	6	63
Creole	½ cup	35	2	51
Lyonnaise	½ cup	60	4	62
w/ butter &				
horseradish	½ cup	100	8	72
Home-style wax				
beans	½ cup	70	2	26
Lima beans & corn				
in cream	½ cup	100	4	36
Lima beans Creole				
(no fat added)	½ cup	60	0	0
Lima beans w/ onions	½ cup	145	4	25
Mexican bean stew	½ cup	105	3	25
Mexican red beans				
w/ pork	½ cup	320	19	53
Pasta e fagioli				
(pasta & beans)	1 cup	300	8	24
Pinto beans	1 cup	240	2	7
Pork & lima beans	1 cup	275	9	29
Red beans & rice				
w/ meat	1 cup	550	19	31
w/o meat	1 cup	315	1	3
Refried beans	½ cup	130	2	14
Shell beans w/ onions	1 cup	65	4	54
Southern green beans	½ cup	35	1	25
Spanish lima beans	1 cup	345	11	28

	AMOUNT	CALORIES	FAT-GRAMS	% FAT
Succotash (lima beans, corn, tomato, bacon)	½ cup	95	3	28
w/ cream		155	6	35
Wax beans in bacon sauce	½ cup	65	3	43
Beets:				
Fresh beets, buttered	½ cup	45	2	42
Harvest beets	½ cup	80	2	22
Hot spiced beets	½ cup	85	2	21
Orange-glazed beets	½ cup	70	2	2
Bok choy (Chinese cabbage):				
Au gratin	½ cup	130	9	62
Fried	½ cup	75	5	60
Oriental-style	½ cup	60	4	58
Steamed	½ cup	10	0	0
Broccoli:				
Broccoli, buttered	3 oz	40	2	43
Broccoli-carrot stir-fry	3 oz	95	6	56
Broccoli Mornay	4 oz	215	15	63
Broccoli Oriental	3 oz	140	8	52
Broccoli soufflé	4 oz	190	13	62
Broccoli steamed	4 oz	25	0	0
Broccoli w/ cheese	3 oz	190	14	66
French-fried broccoli	3 oz	260	16	55
Brussels sprouts:				
buttered	3 oz	45	2	39
in onion cream	3 oz	105	8	69
Polonaise	3 oz	205	23	53
steamed	4 oz	30	0	0

	AMOUNT	CALORIES	FAT-GRAMS	% FAT
Cabbage:				
Bavarian cabbage	½ cup	115	7	55
Cabbage strudel	1	225	18	72
Chinese cabbage				
(bok choy)				
Au gratin	½ cup	130	9	62
Fried	½ cup	75	5	60
Oriental-style	½ cup	60	4	58
Steamed	½ cup	10	0	0
Colcannon				
(Irish cabbage)	6 oz	205	9	40
Country-style				
cabbage	½ cup	115	8	62
Dutch cabbage	½ cup	35	2	49
Escalloped				
cabbage	½ cup	65	3	40
Sauerkraut	½ cup	70	2	26
Sautéed cabbage	½ cup	90	8	79
Carrots:				
Broccoli-carrot				
stir-fry	½ cup	95	6	56
Carrots & celery,				
buttered	½ cup	50	2	36
Carrots Lyonnaise	½ cup	65	3	43
Glazed carrots	½ cup	115	6	46
Peas & carrots	½ cup	85	2	22
Steamed carrots				
Buttered	½ cup	55	2	32
Steamed	½ cup	35	0	0
Turkish carrots	½ cup	175	8	41

	AMOUNT	CALORIES	FAT-GRAMS	% FAT
Cauliflower:				
Au gratin	½ cup	110	7	57
Parmesan	½ cup	75	3	35
Steamed	½ cup	15	0	0
Celery:				
Braised celery	½ cup	30	2	58
Carrots & celery, buttered	½ cup	50	2	36
Peas & celery, buttered	½ cup	70	2	25
Chard, cooked	½ cup	20	0	0
Chinese greens & bean curd in peanut sauce	10 oz	365	19	47
Colach (squash Mexican-style)	6 oz	200	10	45
Colcannon (Irish cabbage)	6 oz	205	9	40
Collard greens, cooked	½ cup	15	0	0
Corn:				
Corn on the cob	1 ear	85	0	0
Buttered	1 ear	120	5	37
Corn pudding	½ cup	135	5	34
Lima beans & corn in cream	½ cup	100	4	36
Mexican corn	½ cup	85	2	21
Succotash	½ cup	95	3	28
Whole-kernel, cooked	½ cup	90	1	10
Crookneck squash soufflé	½ cup	70	4	51
Cucumbers in cream	½ cup	180	18	90
Delmonico potatoes	½ cup	105	3	25
Duchess potatoes	½ cup	155	9	52

	AMOUNT	CALORIES	FAT-GRAMS	% FAT
Dutch cabbage	½ cup	35	2	49
Eggplant:				
Creole	½ cup	40	1	23
Lombardi	1 cup	280	11	35
Parmigiana	1 cup	380	16	38
w/ sherried mushrooms	3 slices	215	6	25
Fresh greens w/ bacon				
drippings	3 oz	90	7	71
Glazed parsnips	3 oz	145	6	37
Green beans	½ cup	20	0	0
& mushrooms				
(no fat added)	½ cup	25	0	0
& water chestnuts	½ cup	65	4	57
Amandine	½ cup	85	6	63
Creole	½ cup	35	2	51
Lyonnaise	½ cup	60	4	62
w/ butter &				
horseradish	½ cup	100	8	72
Home-style wax beans	½ cup	70	2	26
Grilled vegetables	1 serving	240	21	78
Hong Kong spinach	½ cup	70	6	62
Kartoffel Klosse	3 balls	390	16	37
Lettuce	4 leaves	5	0	0
Lima beans & corn				
in cream	½ cup	100	4	36
Lima beans Creole	½ cup	60	0	0
Lima beans w/ onions	½ cup	145	4	25
Lyonnaise potatoes	½ cup	185	7	34
Mexican bean stew	½ cup	105	3	25
Mexican corn	½ cup	85	2	21

	AMOUNT	CALORIES	FAT-GRAMS	% FAT
Mexican red beans				
w/ pork	½ cup	320	19	53
Moravian cabbage	½ cup	190	8	37
Mushrooms:				
Broiled fresh				
mushrooms	½ cup	50	4	70
Sautéed mushrooms	½ cup	45	4	78
O'Brien potatoes	½ cup	165	7	38
Okra, cooked	½ cup	25	0	0
Buttered	½ cup	80	5	56
Onions:				
Fried	½ cup	170	14	75
Fried whole	1 cup	565	39	62
w/ dipping sauce	2 tbsp	710	54	68
Glazed	½ cup	115	6	46
Pearl onions in				
cream sauce	½ cup	150	11	65
Pearl onions, Sarasota	½ cup	85	5	53
Rings	8	275	16	52
Orange-glazed beets	½ cup	70	2	25
Orange-glazed				
sweet potatoes				
(no fat added)	½ cup	130	0	0
Parsnips, glazed	½ cup	145	6	37
Pea pods, steamed	½ cup	25	0	0
Peas:				
Green peas, cooked	½ cup	70	0	0
Buttered	½ cup	105	7	60
Peas & carrots	½ cup	85	2	22
Peas & celery, buttered	½ cup	95	3	28

	AMOUNT	CALORIES	FAT-GRAMS	% FAT
Peas & mushrooms, buttered	½ cup	85	1	14
Peas & onions, buttered	½ cup	100	3	30
Peas & turnips, buttered	½ cup	125	7	50
Stir-fried Chinese pea pods & pepper	½ cup	115	7	55
Peppers:				
Sicilian fried peppers	½ cup	140	10	66
Stir-fried peppers	½ cup	165	13	71
Pinto beans	1 cup	240	2	7
Pork & lima beans	1 cup	275	9	29
Potatoes:				
Baked potato	1 lg	270	0	0
w/ 1 oz bacon	1 lg	350	6	15
w/ 1 oz bacon, sour cream & chives	1 lg	480	16	30
w/ 1 tbsp butter	1 lg	370	11	27
w/ butter, bacon, sour cream & chives	1 lg	580	22	34
w/ cheese & bacon	1 lg	760	26	31
w/ cheese & broccoli	1 lg	760	26	31
w/ chili & cheese	1 lg	700	23	29
w/ ¼ cup sour cream	1 lg	400	11	24
Baked potato skins w/ cheese	¼ potato	60	3	29
Boiled potatoes, buttered	½ cup	125	3	22
Cheese fries	1 cup	595	38	57
w/ ranch dressing	2 tbsp	750	54	66

	AMOUNT	CALORIES	FAT-GRAMS	% FAT
Cottage fries	½ cup	185	7	34
Creamed potatoes	½ cup	105	2	17
Delmonico potatoes	½ cup	105	3	25
Escalloped potatoes	½ cup	115	3	23
French fries	1 reg serving	235	12	46
	1 lg serving	355	19	48
Fried potato skins	¼ potato	55	3	50
Hash browns	½ cup	163	11	61
Home-fried potatoes	½ cup	220	8	33
Hot potato salad	1 cup	250	16	58
Kartoffel Klosse	3 balls	390	16	37
Lyonnaise potatoes	½ cup	185	7	34
Mashed or whipped potatoes	½ cup	125	3	29
O'Brien potatoes	½ cup	165	7	38
Oven-roasted potatoes	1 med potato	210	11	47
Potato cake Parmesan	½ cup	170	7	37
Potato chips	1 oz	150	10	60
Chef-prepared	1 potato	285	14	44
Potato dumplings	2	145	1	6
Potatoes au gratin	½ cup	200	11	49
Potatoes Champs Elysées	9 oz	350	20	51
Potatoes Hongroise	6 oz	140	4	26
Potatoes Lorette	7 oz	685	45	59
Potatoes Theresa	1 cup	170	3	16
Potato gnocchi	5 oz	210	6	26

	AMOUNT	CALORIES	FAT-GRAMS	% FAT
Potato pancakes	1 cake	495	13	24
Potato patty	1	255	16	56
Potato puffs	2	165	5	27
Potato slices (skin on)	1 potato	240	14	52
Potato wedges (skin on)	1 potato	240	14	52
Rissole potatoes	½ cup	200	11	49
Seasoned/coated fries	1 potato	305	12	35
Shoestring potatoes	1 potato	285	14	44
Spiral fries	1 potato	285	14	44
Stuffed potato	1 sm	180	5	25
Sweet potatoes.				
See separate entry.				
Ratatouille	1 cup	145	10	62
Rutabagas	½ cup	30	0	0
Buttered	½ cup	50	2	36
Sauerkraut	½ cup	70	2	26
Spinach:				
Hong Kong spinach (sautéed spinach, Oriental soy sauce)	½ cup	70	5	62
Spinach w/ bacon drippings	½ cup	90	7	71
Spinach, buttered	½ cup	55	2	33
Spinach soufflé	½ cup	145	9	57
Steamed spinach	½ cup	20	0	0
Wilted spinach	½ cup	130	11	76
Squash:				
Baked acorn squash	½ squash	165	4	22
Baked crookneck squash	½ cup	20	1	50

	AMOUNT	CALORIES	FAT-GRAMS	% FAT
Baked squash (butter, brown sugar)	1 pc	75	4	47
Colach (squash Mexican-style)	6 oz	200	10	45
Crookneck squash, buttered	½ cup	35	2	51
Whipped fresh winter squash	½ cup	80	2	22
Zucchini à la Française	5 oz	120	6	45
Zucchini & tomatoes	½ cup	40	2	43
Zucchini fritters	2	76	6	71
Zucchini Neapolitan	½ cup	140	12	76
Shell beans w/ onions	1 cup	65	4	54
Sicilian fried peppers	½ cup	140	10	66
Spanish lima beans	1 cup	345	11	28
Stewed tomatoes	½ cup	55	2	31
Succotash	½ cup	95	3	28
Sweet potatoes:				
Candied sweet potatoes	½ cup	205	2	9
Escalloped sweet potato & apple	½ cup	145	3	19
Mashed or whipped sweet potato	½ cup	135	4	26
Orange-glazed sweet potatoes	½ cup	130	0	0
Sweet potatoes w/ pecans	½ cup	240	5	19
Tomatoes:				
Baked or broiled tomatoes	½ cup	30	1	31

	AMOUNT	CALORIES	FAT-GRAMS	% FAT
Baked stuffed tomato	1	55	1	16
Escalloped tomatoes	½ cup	115	5	39
Pan-fried tomatoes	½ cup	290	21	65
Stewed tomatoes	½ cup	55	2	31
Tomatoes & celery	½ cup	30	0	0
Tomatoes & okra	½ cup	55	2	33
Turkish carrots	½ cup	175	8	41
Turnips	½ cup	15	0	0
Buttered	½ cup	10	0	0
Swedish-style	½ cup	190	10	47
Wax beans in bacon sauce	½ cup	65	3	43
Vegetable medley	1 cup	100	4	35
Vegetables, creamed	½ cup	60	2	30
Vegetables amandine	½ cup	60	3	43
Vegetables au gratin	½ cup	90	6	59
Vegetables Hollandaise	½ cup	215	21	88
Vegetables Macedoine	½ cup	80	4	45
Vegetables Oriental	½ cup	35	3	82
Vegetable stir-fry w/ bean curd	1 cup	180	13	65
Veggie fajita wrap	1	460	23	45
Yams, baked	½ cup	80	0	0
Zucchini:				
& tomatoes	½ cup	40	2	43
à la Française	5 oz	120	6	45
Cooked	½ cup	15	0	0
Fritters	2	75	6	72
Neapolitan	½ cup	140	12	76

VEGETARIAN ENTRÉES

	AMOUNT	CALORIES	FAT-GRAMS	% FAT
Asparagus à la Polonaise (asparagus, egg, cream sauce, buttered crumbs)	1 cup	205	11	48
Avocado burgers:				
w/ bun	8 oz	565	30	48
w/o bun	8 oz	435	28	58
Bean burgers:				
w/ bun	8 oz	700	42	54
w/o bun	8 oz	570	40	63
Bean burrito	1	400	6	13
w/ sour cream		450	12	24
Bean curd & vegetable stir-fry	1 cup	180	13	65
Bean curd in peanut sauce w/ Chinese greens	10 oz	365	19	47
Black bean enchilada	1	445	20	41
Brown rice w/ peas, onions & Parmesan	1 cup	320	10	28
Brown vegetable rice	1 cup	370	24	58

	AMOUNT	CALORIES	FAT-GRAMS	% FAT
Calcutta medley (soybeans, bulgur & brown rice w/ peanuts, apple, yogurt, curry)	1 cup	860	33	34
California casserole (brown rice, sour cream, cottage cheese, green chilies, cheddar)	1 cup	550	38	62
Chalupas (beans, tortilla, cheese, avocado, salsa)	2 sm	325	18	50
Cheese & nut loaf (brown rice, cottage cheese, sesame seeds, peanuts, walnuts, wheat germ, eggs)	1 cup	525	42	72
Cheese enchilada	1	490	34	62
Chili relleno	1	340	24	64
Cottage cheese patties (cottage cheese, wheat germ, bread crumbs, walnuts, cream of mushroom soup)	2	440	30	62
Couscous w/ fruit	1 cup	450	16	32
Crusty Soybean Crowd-Pleaser (soybeans, corn, tomatoes, onion, wheat germ, Parmesan, brown rice)	1 cup	205	11	33

	AMOUNT	CALORIES	FAT-GRAMS	% FAT
Curried soybeans & peanuts over brown rice	1 cup	490	15	28
Curried stuffed pepper (millet, lentils, peas, mushrooms, carrots, almonds, cashews)	1	585	34	52
Dilled carrot cutlets (soybeans, carrots, peanuts, wheat germ, oil)	1 cup	355	23	58
East-West bean bake (brown rice, soybeans, wheat germ, mozzarella)	1 cup	265	13	49
Eggplant & cheese casserole	1 cup	215	14	58
Eggplant bake	1 cup	420	12	25
Eggs Grinnel (egg, spinach, cheese)	1 egg	215	15	62
Esau's Potage (brown rice, lentils, onions, celery, mushrooms)	1 cup	410	15	33
Falafel patties, broiled	8 oz	300	15	45
Golden parsley potatoes (potatoes, cottage cheese, cheddar)	1 cup	285	13	41
Leafy Chinese tofu (tofu, spinach, peanut oil)	1 cup	220	17	70

	AMOUNT	CALORIES	FAT-GRAMS	% FAT
Legumes Continental (garbanzo beans, pinto beans, cabbage, cheddar)	1 cup	795	54	61
Mexican bean stew	1 cup	220	4	16
Peanut sauce over vegetable salad	1 serving	778	64	62
Potato-bean bake (lentils, soybeans, mashed potatoes, mushrooms)	10 oz	440	22	45
Potatoes Gruyère	8 oz	365	19	47
Potato pancakes	2 cakes	495	13	24
Quesadilla (6")	1	245	16	58
Red & sweet curried rice	8 oz	445	13	26
Russian Surprise (navy beans, potatoes, onions, cucumber, sour cream, pumpernickel)	8 oz	520	20	35
Russian sweet cabbage	12 oz	325	10	28
Sesame vegetable rice (4 oz rice, 8 oz vegetables)	12 oz	545	29	48
Soybean souffle	8 oz	135	9	60
Spinach-rice pot	8 oz	580	42	65
Spinach & tomato casserole	8 oz	135	7	46
Stuffed eggplant	1 slice	305	23	68

	AMOUNT	CALORIES	FAT-GRAMS	% FAT
Summer squash & brown rice (w/ yogurt, Parmesan, egg, bread crumbs)	8 oz	230	14	54
Tostada w/ avocado	1	590	37	56
Vegetable paella	8 oz	635	23	32
Vegetable stew	8 oz	505	32	57
Veggie burger				
w/ bun	6 oz	355	18	46
w/o bun	6 oz	225	16	64
Veggie wrapper	1	840	54	58
Walnut-rice cheddar loaf	8 oz	590	42	64
Zucchini & cheddar casserole	8 oz	325	18	50
Zucchini bake	8 oz	105	5	43
Zucchini frittata	2 eggs	215	16	67
Zucchini-rice bake	8 oz	195	11	50

FAST-FOOD RESTAURANTS

Most of the foods offered at fast-food restaurants are rich in fat, so it makes good sense to visit these restaurants infrequently if reducing fat is a concern.

When you do choose to eat fast food, be aware of a dangerous trend: portion sizes and fat content have recently spun out of control. Because of America's addiction to "bigness," size has become a marketing device and often equated with better value, i.e., "getting more for less." Witness "Biggie" fries, double or triple burgers, and giant soft drinks. And Burger King's offer of a Double Supreme Cheeseburger, along with large fries and a medium drink, for under $3. It's why McDonald's can promote two Big Macs for less than $2. And burger chains are not alone. Everyone is serving larger portions . . . pizza, soft drinks, chicken. A gargantuan Macho Meal at Del Taco weighs more than 4 pounds!

In addition, the fat content of many fast foods has skyrocketed. Cheese and bacon are routinely added to a long line of items. If you order the Triple Decker pizza at Pizza Hut, for instance, you'll get more fat than you would from a stick and a half of butter!

Smarter, low-fat choices *do* exist at fast-food restaurants, but you need to look for them before you order. That's how this guide can help.

GENERAL TIPS

- Make smart choices. The fast-food industry has responded to public pressure by offering some lower-fat items. (Remember, there are very few fast-food items that are truly low in fat, but lower-fat items do exist.) Arby's has the Light Roast Deluxe Chicken Sandwich with just 6 grams of fat, slightly more than the Turkey Breast Sandwich at Boston Market

(4 grams of fat). And a regular hamburger at Burger King has just 15 grams of fat. But the Double Western Bacon Cheeseburger at Carl's Jr. has 63 grams of fat and 1,030 calories. And the Taco Salad with shell and dressing at Taco Bell has 87 grams of fat and 1,170 calories. Each provides more fat in a single meal than most people should consume in an entire day.

- Watch out for added fat such as bacon, cheese, "special sauce," mayonnaise and salad dressings. A salad is a healthy food, but it can be turned into an unhealthy choice with added fat. A prepackaged salad with chicken has only about 3 or 4 grams of fat. But top it with a packet of ranch dressing at Burger King, and you'll add about 37 grams of fat. It's a far better idea to ask for diet or no-oil dressings. McDonald's Fat-Free Herb Vinaigrette, for instance, contains no fat.

- When ordering breakfast, opt for pancakes and syrup (without butter or margarine) instead of breakfast sandwiches that combine cheese, egg and/or meat filling with a muffin, croissant or biscuit. This switch saves about 30 grams of fat. Watch out for French Toast Sticks. An order at Burger King contains 27 grams of fat.

- Pizza can be a good bet if you order wisely. Pass up fatty meat toppings such as pepperoni, ground beef and sausage, which drive up the fat content to the level of a cheeseburger. Order cheese pizza "with half the cheese, extra tomato sauce and more vegetables," and you'll have a fast food you can live with.

- At Mexican fast-food outlets, order the plain bean burrito or tostada for less fat than the loaded versions. Look for light versions such as Taco Time's Soft Chicken Taco—it's just 8 grams of fat.

- Think about preparation methods. The biggest problem is that most fast foods are fried, which means added fat.

SOME SMARTER CHOICES	CALORIES	FAT-GRAMS	%FAT
Hardee's Pancakes (3)	280	2	6
Long John Silver's Flavorbaked Fish (1 serving)	90	3	28
Boston Market ¼ chicken, white meat, w/o skin & wing	160	4	22
Dairy Queen/Brazier BBQ Beef Sandwich	225	4	16
Subway 6" Turkey Breast & Ham Sub	295	5	15
Arby's Light Roast Turkey Deluxe Sandwich	260	6	21
Taco Bell Light Bean Burrito	330	6	16
Wendy's Chili (small size)	220	7	29
KFC BBQ Chicken Sandwich	255	8	28
Jack in the Box Chicken Fajita Pita	280	9	29
McDonald's Regular Hamburger	260	9	31
Domino's 12" Cheese Pizza, Hand Tossed (2 slices)	350	11	28

HAMBURGERS

Hamburgers are still America's favorite fast food. But not all hamburgers are the same, as shown in the table that follows:

HAMBURGER	CALORIES	FAT-GRAMS	%FAT
Wendy's Single, plain	360	16	40
McDonald's Quarter Pounder	420	21	44
McDonald's Big Mac	560	31	50
Wendy's Big Bacon Classic	580	30	47
Hardee's "The Boss" Burger	570	33	52
Burger King Big King	600	36	54
Burger King Whopper	640	39	55
Burger King Double Whopper w/ Cheese	960	63	59
Jack in the Box Ultimate Cheeseburger	1,030	79	69

- As size and number of patties increase, so does the fat. Single hamburgers have about 2 ounces of meat, quarter-pounders about 3 ounces, and triples have 4 or more ounces. Order items identified as "small," "single" or "junior." Avoid those labeled "jumbo," "super," "double," "triple," "extra-large" and "big."

- Don't make the mistake of eating too many small burgers. There is no advantage in eating two Wendy's

Junior hamburgers with a combined 20 grams of fat, for instance, over one Wendy's regular hamburger at 16 grams.

- Watch out for fatty add-ons. Opt for a plain hamburger with lettuce, tomato, onion and ketchup (10 to 15 grams of fat) instead of the supreme version loaded with cheese, bacon, mayonnaise or mayo-based "special sauces" (50 to 60 grams of fat).

FRIED FOODS

- Fried chicken is extremely high in fat. One-half chicken with skin at Kenny Rogers Roasters has 28 grams of fat, while KFC's "Hot & Spicy" breast has 35 grams. When you eat fried chicken, choose the breast and remove the skin and breading. Exercise portion control. Many of the complements are high in fat, such as coleslaw, onion rings and French fries.

- Chicken nuggets are battered and fried, so most of their calories come from fat. Six McDonald's McNuggets yield about 17 grams of fat, while three Spicy Buffalo Crispy Strips at KFC have 19.

- Fried fish and seafood have the same basic problem as fried chicken. Avoid deep-fried fish, oysters, scallops, shrimp and clams. Unfortunately, fried seafood usually comes with high-fat side dishes such as coleslaw or French fries. A good example is the Fish, Shrimp & Clams Dinner (w/ fries, hush puppies and coleslaw) at Long John Silver's with 70 grams of fat. Instead, choose low-fat items such as Long John Silver's Flavorbaked Fish & Chicken (1 piece each) over Rice (w/ baked potato and green beans). The cost to your budget is only 10 grams of fat.

- A typical medium serving of French fries has 17 grams of fat. Some chains offer baked potatoes with steamed vegetables as a low-fat alternative.

SANDWICHES

- Roast beef sandwiches can be a good alternative to hamburgers. Stick with the regular or junior-size sandwich, and avoid high-fat extras such as mayonnaise, mayo-based sauces and cheese.

- Avoid croissant sandwiches. Many croissants contain the fat equivalent of four pats of butter.

- Many delis offer extra-lean corned beef, pastrami and beef brisket, but watch out for portion size. Sandwiches can be large enough to feed two people, so order a half-sandwich or split it with a friend. Also, be careful with side dishes such as creamy coleslaw and potato salad.

- High-fat sub sandwiches are those made with bologna, hard or Genoa salami, pepperoni, mortadella and cheese. Opt instead for turkey, smoked turkey, ham and lean roast beef. Avoid oil and mayonnaise in favor of mustard, onions, lettuce, pickles and hot peppers.

- Stick with low-fat sandwich fillers such

as roasted turkey breast, roasted or grilled chicken breast, lean roast beef and lean ham. Avoid cold cuts, tuna or chicken with mayonnaise, egg salad, cheese sandwiches and cheese melts.

- The best choice for a chicken sandwich is a skinless, grilled breast. Watch out for sandwiches that use fried chicken— Jack in the Box's Really Big Chicken Sandwich has 56 grams of fat, while their Chicken Fajita Pita has just 9. As with other sandwiches, cut out the extras such as mayonnaise, mayo-based sauces, cheese and cheese sauces.

- A fried fish fillet sandwich is not a good choice. Breaded, fried in grease and covered with mayonnaise and fatty sauces, it is an item to be avoided. Skipper's Double Create A Catch Sandwich, for example, will set you back over 70 fat-grams.

- Watch out for fatty condiments. A Subway 6-inch Roast Beef Sandwich without oil has about 5 grams of fat; with oil, it has 25 grams. Use mustard, horseradish or ketchup to moisten the sandwich, but skip oil, butter, margarine and mayonnaise.

FAST-FOOD RESTAURANTS

	AMOUNT	CALORIES	FAT-GRAMS	% FAT
ARBY'S				
BREAKFAST ITEMS				
Bacon	I serving	90	7	70
Biscuits				
Plain	I	280	15	48
Bacon	I	320	18	51
Ham	I	325	17	47
Sausage	I	460	32	62
Croissants				
Plain	I	220	12	49
Bacon & Egg	I	430	30	63
Ham & Cheese	I	345	21	54
Mushroom/Cheese	I	495	38	69
Sausage & Egg	I	520	39	68
Danish, Cinnamon Nut	I	360	11	28
Eggs	I serving	95	8	76
French Toastix	I serving	430	21	44
Maple Syrup	I serving	120	0	0
Ham	I serving	45	1	20
Muffin, Blueberry	I	230	9	35
Platters				
Bacon	I serving	595	33	50
Egg	I serving	460	24	47

	AMOUNT	CALORIES	FAT-GRAMS	% FAT
Ham	1 serving	520	26	46
Sausage	1 serving	640	41	58
Sausage	1 serving	165	15	82

DESSERTS

Cheese Cake	1	320	23	65
Chocolate Chip Cookie	1	125	6	43
Polar Swirls				
Butterfinger	1	460	18	36
Heath	1	545	22	36
Oreo	1	480	20	37
Peanut Butter Cup	1	515	24	42
Snickers	1	510	19	33
Turnovers				
Apple	1	330	14	38
Cherry	1	320	13	36

DRINKS & SHAKES

Drinks

Coffee	8 oz	0	0	0
Hot Chocolate	8 oz	110	1	10
Iced Tea	16 oz	5	0	0
Milk, 2%	8 oz	120	4	33
Orange Juice	6 oz	80	0	0
Soft Drinks (12 oz)				
Coca-Cola Classic	1	140	0	0
Diet Coke	1	0	0	0
Nehi Orange	1	190	0	0

	AMOUNT	CALORIES	FAT-GRAMS	% FAT
Pepsi Cola	1	160	0	0
R.C. Cola	1	175	0	0
R.C. Diet Rite	1	0	0	0
R.C. Root Beer	1	175	0	0
7-Up	1	145	0	0
Diet 7-Up	1	5	0	0
Upper Ten	1	170	0	0
Shakes				
Chocolate	1	450	12	23
Jamocha	1	385	10	23
Vanilla	1	360	12	30
POTATOES				
Baked, Plain	1	355	0	0
Broccoli & Cheddar	1	570	20	31
w/ Margarine &				
Sour Cream	1	580	24	37
Deluxe	1	735	36	44
French Fries				
Cheddar Fries	1 serving	335	18	49
Curly Fries	1 serving	300	15	45
Homestyle Fries				
Small	1 serving	210	10	43
Medium	1 serving	340	16	42
Large	1 serving	425	19	40
Hash Brown				
Nuggets	1 serving	270	17	57
Potato Cakes	1 serving	205	12	53

	AMOUNT	CALORIES	FAT-GRAMS	% FAT
SALADS & SALAD DRESSINGS				
Salads				
Chef's	1	205	10	42
Garden	1	120	5	40
Roast Chicken	1	205	7	32
Side	1	25	0	0
Croutons	1 serving	60	2	34
Salad Dressings				
Blue Cheese	1 serving	290	31	96
Buttermilk Ranch, Reduced-Calorie	1 serving	50	0	0
Honey French	1 serving	280	23	74
Italian, Reduced-Calorie	1 serving	20	1	45
Red Ranch	1 serving	75	6	72
Thousand Island	1 serving	260	26	90
SANDWICHES				
Chicken				
Breaded Fillet	1	535	28	46
Cordon Bleu	1	625	33	47
Grilled Barbecue	1	390	13	30
Grilled Deluxe	1	430	20	42
Light Roast Deluxe	1	275	6	22
Roast Club	1	545	31	50
Roast Deluxe	1	435	22	46
Roast Santa Fe	1	435	22	43
Fish Fillet	1	530	27	46
Ham 'N Cheese	1	360	14	35
Ham 'N Cheese Melt	1	330	13	36

	AMOUNT	CALORIES	FAT-GRAMS	% FAT
Roast Beef				
Arby's Melt w/ Cheddar	1	370	18	43
Arby Q	1	430	18	37
Bac'n Cheddar Deluxe	1	540	34	57
Beef'n Cheddar	1	510	28	49
Big Montana	1	685	35	46
Giant	1	555	28	45
Junior	1	325	14	39
Light Deluxe	1	180	10	50
Regular	1	390	19	44
Super	1	525	27	46
Roast Turkey,				
Light Deluxe	1	260	7	21
Sub Roll Sandwiches				
French Dip	1	475	22	41
Hot Ham 'N Swiss	1	500	23	41
Italian Sub	1	635	36	51
Philly Beef 'N Swiss	1	755	47	55
Roast Beef Sub	1	700	42	54
Triple Cheese Melt	1	720	45	55
Turkey Sub	1	550	27	44
SAUCES				
Arby's Sauce	1 serving	15	0	0
Barbecue Sauce	1 serving	30	0	0
Beef Stock Au Jus Sauce	1 serving	10	0	0
Cheddar Cheese Sauce	1 serving	35	3	77
Honey Mayonnaise, Reduced-Calorie	1 serving	70	7	90

	AMOUNT	CALORIES	FAT-GRAMS	% FAT
Horsey Sauce	I serving	60	5	75
Italian Sub Sauce	I serving	70	7	90
Ketchup	I serving	15	0	0
Mayonnaise	I serving	110	12	100
Light	I serving	15	1	75
Mustard	I serving	5	0	0
Parmesan Cheese				
Sauce	I serving	70	7	90
Tartar Sauce	I serving	140	15	96

SOUPS

Boston Clam Chowder	I serving	190	9	42
Cheese	I serving	280	18	58
Chicken Noodle	I serving	80	2	22
Chili	I serving	220	10	41
Cream of Broccoli	I serving	160	8	45
Mixed Vegetables	I serving	90	4	40
Potato w/ Bacon	I serving	170	7	37

ARTHUR TREACHER'S

CHICKEN

Patties	2	370	22	53
Sandwich	I	415	19	42

FISH

Cod Fillet	I serving	245	14	52
Fried Fish	2 pieces	355	20	50
Sandwich	I	440	24	49
Shrimp	7 pieces	380	24	58

	AMOUNT	CALORIES	FAT-GRAMS	% FAT
OTHER ITEMS				
Coleslaw	1 serving	125	8	60
French Fries, Chips	1 serving	275	13	43
Hushpuppy	1	205	15	66

AU BON PAIN

BREAKFAST ITEMS				
Bagels				
Plain	1	380	2	5
Cinnamon	1	395	2	5
Onion	1	390	2	5
Sesame	1	425	5	11
Croissants				
Plain	1	220	10	41
Almond	1	420	25	54
Apple	1	250	10	36
Blueberry Cheese	1	380	20	47
Chocolate	1	400	24	54
Cinnamon Raisin	1	390	13	30
Coconut Pecan	1	440	23	47
Hazelnut Chocolate	1	480	28	53
Raspberry Cheese	1	400	20	45
Strawberry Cheese	1	400	20	45
Sweet Cheese	1	420	23	49
Danish Pastry				
Cheese	1	390	22	51
Cherry	1	335	16	43
Cherry Dumpling	1	360	13	33
Raspberry	1	335	16	43

	AMOUNT	CALORIES	FAT-GRAMS	% FAT
Hot Croissants				
Ham & Cheese	1	370	20	49
Spinach & Cheese	1	290	16	50
Turkey & Cheddar	1	410	22	48
Turkey & Havarti	1	410	21	46
Muffins				
Blueberry	1	390	4	9
Bran	1	390	11	25
Carrot	1	450	22	44
Corn	1	460	17	33
Cranberry Walnut	1	350	13	33
Oat Bran Apple	1	400	2	5
Pumpkin	1	410	16	35
Whole Grain	1	440	16	35
BREADS & ROLLS				
Breads				
Baguette	1 loaf	810	2	2
Cheese	1 loaf	1,670	29	16
Four-Grain	1 loaf	1,420	11	7
Onion Herb	1 loaf	1,430	13	8
Pita Pocket	2 slices	80	0	0
Ponsienne	1 loaf	1,490	4	2
Sandwich				
Multi-grain	2 slices	390	3	7
Rye	2 slices	375	4	10
Rolls				
Alpine	1	220	3	12
Country Seed	1	220	4	16

	AMOUNT	CALORIES	FAT-GRAMS	% FAT
Health	1	250	2	7
Petit Pan	1	220	0	0
Pumpernickel	1	210	2	9
Rye	1	230	2	8
Sandwich				
Braided	1	390	11	26
Croissant	1	300	14	42
French	1	320	0	0
Hearth	1	370	3	7
Soft	1	310	8	23
3-Seed Raisin	1	250	4	14
Vegetable	1	230	5	20

COOKIES

	AMOUNT	CALORIES	FAT-GRAMS	% FAT
Chocolate Chip	1	280	15	48
Chocolate Chunk Pecan	1	290	17	53
White Chocolate	1	300	17	51
Oatmeal Raisin	1	250	9	32
Peanut Butter	1	290	15	47
Shortbread	1	425	26	55

SALADS & SALAD DRESSINGS

Salads

	AMOUNT	CALORIES	FAT-GRAMS	% FAT
Cracked Pepper Chicken	1 serving	100	2	18
Grilled Chicken	1 serving	110	2	16
Tarragon Chicken	1 serving	310	15	44
Green				
Small	1 serving	20	0	0
Large	1 serving	40	0	0
Tuna	1 serving	350	25	64
Shrimp	1 serving	100	2	18

	AMOUNT	CALORIES	FAT-GRAMS	% FAT
Salad Dressing				
Italian, Low-Calorie	1 serving	70	6	79

SANDWICHES & WRAPS

Sandwiches

	AMOUNT	CALORIES	FAT-GRAMS	% FAT
Cracked Pepper Chicken				
on French Roll	1	440	3	6
on Hearth Roll	1	490	5	9
on Soft Roll	1	430	10	21
Grilled Chicken				
on French Roll	1	450	5	10
on Hearth Roll	1	500	7	13
on Soft Roll	1	440	12	25
Tarragon Chicken				
on French Roll	1	590	16	24
on Hearth Roll	1	640	18	25
on Soft Roll	1	580	23	36
Ham Sandwich				
on French Roll	1	470	8	15
on Hearth Roll	1	520	10	17
on Soft Roll	1	460	15	29
Roast Beef Sandwich				
on French Roll	1	500	9	16
on Hearth Roll	1	550	11	18
on Soft Roll	1	490	16	29
Turkey Sandwich				
on French Roll	1	420	2	4
on Hearth Roll	1	470	4	8
on Soft Roll	1	410	9	20

	AMOUNT	CALORIES	FAT-GRAMS	% FAT
Wraps				
Chicken Caesar Wrap	1	630	31	44
Southwestern Tuna Wrap	1	950	64	60
Summer Turkey Wrap	1	550	12	20
SANDWICH FILLINGS, CHEESE				
Boursin	1 serving	290	29	90
Brie	1 serving	300	24	72
Cheddar	1 serving	110	9	74
Provolone	1 serving	155	13	73
Swiss	1 serving	330	24	65
SOUPS, CHILI & POT PIE				
Soups				
Beef Barley	1 cup	75	2	24
	1 bowl	110	3	24
Chicken Noodle	1 cup	80	1	11
	1 bowl	120	2	13
Clam Chowder	1 cup	290	18	56
	1 bowl	435	27	56
Cream of Broccoli	1 cup	200	17	76
	1 bowl	300	26	77
Minestrone	1 cup	105	2	17
Split Pea	1 cup	175	1	5
	1 bowl	265	2	7
Tomato	1 cup	60	1	15
	1 bowl	90	2	17
Vegetarian	1 cup	30	0	0
	1 bowl	45	0	0

AU BON PAIN

	AMOUNT	CALORIES	FAT-GRAMS	% FAT
CHILI				
Vegetarian	1 cup	140	3	19
	1 bowl	210	4	17
POT PIE				
Chicken	1 serving	440	21	43

BASKIN-ROBBINS

	AMOUNT	CALORIES	FAT-GRAMS	% FAT
CONES				
Sugar	1	60	1	15
Waffle	1	140	2	13
ICE CREAM, REGULAR DELUXE				
Banana Nut	½ cup	140	9	58
Banana Strawberry	½ cup	130	6	42
Baseball Nut	½ cup	150	8	43
Black Walnut	½ cup	150	10	60
Blueberry Cheesecake	½ cup	150	7	42
Butterfinger	½ cup	160	8	45
	1 scoop	300	15	45
Caramel Chocolate Crunch	½ cup	160	9	51
Cherry Cheesecake	½ cup	150	7	42
Cherries Jubilee	½ cup	130	6	42
	1 scoop	240	11	42
Chewy Baby Ruth	½ cup	160	9	51
Chocolate	½ cup	150	8	43
	1 scoop	270	14	47
Chocolate Almond	½ cup	170	10	53
	1 scoop	300	18	54

	AMOUNT	CALORIES	FAT-GRAMS	% FAT
Chocolate Chip	½ cup	150	9	54
	I scoop	260	15	52
Choc Chip Cookie Dough	½ cup	170	10	53
Chocolate Fudge	½ cup	160	9	51
	I scoop	290	15	47
Choc Mousse Royale	½ cup	170	9	48
	I scoop	320	16	45
Chocolate Ribbon	½ cup	140	7	45
Chunks 'N Chips	½ cup	160	9	51
Chunky Heath Bar	½ cup	170	9	48
Cinnamon Tax Crunch	½ cup	160	8	40
Cookies 'N Cream	½ cup	160	9	51
	I scoop	280	17	55
French Vanilla	½ cup	160	11	62
	I scoop	280	18	58
Fudge Brownie	½ cup	170	10	53
	I scoop	320	18	51
German Chocolate Cake	½ cup	170	11	58
	I scoop	310	15	44
Gold Medal Ribbon	½ cup	140	7	45
Here Comes the Fudge	½ cup	150	7	42
Jamoca	½ cup	130	7	48
	I scoop	240	13	49
Jamoca Almond Fudge	½ cup	150	8	48
	I scoop	270	14	47
Lemon Custard	½ cup	140	7	45
Mint Choc Chip	½ cup	150	9	54
	I scoop	260	15	52

	AMOUNT	CALORIES	FAT-GRAMS	% FAT
New York Cheesecake	½ cup	150	9	54
Nutty Coconut	½ cup	170	11	58
Old Fashioned				
Peanut Butter	½ cup	160	10	56
	1 scoop	280	18	58
Oregon Blackberry	½ cup	130	7	48
	1 scoop	230	12	47
Peach	½ cup	130	6	42
	1 scoop	230	11	43
Peanut Butter 'N Choc	½ cup	180	11	55
	1 scoop	330	20	55
Pink Bubble Gum	½ cup	150	7	42
Pistachio-Almond	½ cup	160	11	62
	1 scoop	290	18	5
Pralines 'n Cream	½ cup	160	8	45
	1 scoop	280	14	45
Pumpkin Pie	½ cup	130	6	42
Quarterback Crunch	½ cup	160	9	51
Rocky Road	½ cup	160	8	45
	scoop	300	14	42
Rum Raisin	½ cup	140	6	39
S'Mores	½ cup	170	8	42
	1 scoop	300	13	39
Strawberry Cheesecake	½ cup	150	7	42
	1 scoop	260	13	45
Strawberry Shortcake	½ cup	150	8	48
S'Crunchous Crunch	½ cup	170	8	42
Triple Chocolate Passion	½ cup	180	10	50
Vanilla	½ cup	140	8	51
	1 scoop	240	14	53

	AMOUNT	CALORIES	FAT-GRAMS	% FAT
Very Berry Strawberry	½ cup	120	6	45
	1 scoop	220	10	41
Winter White Chocolate	½ cup	150	8	48
World Class Chocolate	½ cup	150	8	48
	1 scoop	280	14	45

ICE CREAM, LIGHT

	AMOUNT	CALORIES	FAT-GRAMS	% FAT
Almond Buttercrunch	½ cup	120	4	30
Chocolate Caramel Nut	½ cup	130	4	28
Double Raspberry	½ cup	90	2	20
Espresso & Cream	½ cup	110	4	33
Praline Dream	½ cup	120	4	30
Rocky Path	½ cup	130	4	28

ICE CREAM, FAT-FREE

	AMOUNT	CALORIES	FAT-GRAMS	% FAT
Caramel Ban Surprise	½ cup	110	0	0
Chocolate Marshmallow	½ cup	110	0	0
Chocolate Vanilla Twist	½ cup	100	0	0
Chocolate Wonder	½ cup	90	0	0
Jamoca Swirl	½ cup	110	0	0
Just Peachy	½ cup	100	0	0
Peanut Butter Cream	½ cup	90	0	0

ICE CREAM, NO SUGAR ADDED

	AMOUNT	CALORIES	FAT-GRAMS	% FAT
Berries 'N Banana	½ cup	80	1	11
Cherry Cordial	½ cup	100	2	18
Chocolate Chip	½ cup	100	3	27
Chocolate Choc Chip	½ cup	100	3	27
Chunky Banana	½ cup	90	2	20

	AMOUNT	CALORIES	FAT-GRAMS	% FAT
Coconut Fudge	½ cup	110	2	16
Jamoca Swiss Almond	½ cup	100	3	27
Pineapple Coconut	½ cup	90	2	20
Raspberry Revelation	½ cup	100	1	18
Thin Mint	½ cup	100	3	27
Vanilla Swiss Almond	½ cup	110	2	16

ICE CREAM BAR

	AMOUNT	CALORIES	FAT-GRAMS	% FAT
Chocolate	1 bar	150	5	30

ICES, SHERBETS & SORBETS

	AMOUNT	CALORIES	FAT-GRAMS	% FAT
Daiquiri Ice	½ cup	110	0	0
	1 scoop	140	0	0
Grape Ice	½ cup	110	0	0
Margarita Ice	½ cup	110	0	0
Rainbow Sherbet	½ cup	120	2	15
	1 scoop	160	2.5	14
Orange Sherbet	½ cup	120	2	15
	1 scoop	160	2.5	14
Red Raspberry Sorbet	½ cup	120	0	0
	1 scoop	140	0	0

YOGURT, FROZEN, LOW-FAT

	AMOUNT	CALORIES	FAT-GRAMS	% FAT
Blueberry	½ cup	120	2	15
Cheesecake	½ cup	120	2	15
Chocolate	½ cup	120	2	15
Vanilla	½ cup	120	2	15

	AMOUNT	CALORIES	FAT-GRAMS	% FAT

YOGURT, FROZEN, NONFAT

	AMOUNT	CALORIES	FAT-GRAMS	% FAT
Black Cherry	½ cup	110	0	0
Chocolate Mint	½ cup	100	0	0
Dutch Chocolate	½ cup	100	0	0
Kahlúa	½ cup	100	0	0
Key Lime	½ cup	100	0	0
Maple Walnut	½ cup	100	0	0
Peach	½ cup	100	0	0
Peppermint Twist	½ cup	100	0	0
Raspberry	½ cup	100	0	0
Strawberry	½ cup	100	0	0
Vanilla	½ cup	110	0	0

YOGURT, FROZEN, FAT-FREE/SUGAR-REDUCED

	AMOUNT	CALORIES	FAT-GRAMS	% FAT
Apple Pie	½ cup	80	0	0
Cafe Mocha	½ cup	80	0	0
Chocolate	½ cup	80	0	0
Vanilla	½ cup	80	0	0
Whata Banana	½ cup	80	0	0

TOPPINGS

	AMOUNT	CALORIES	FAT-GRAMS	% FAT
Butterscotch	2 oz	200	2	9
Hot Fudge	1 oz	100	3	2
No Sugar Added	1 oz	90	0	0
Praline Caramel	1 oz	90	0	0
Strawberry	1 oz	60	0	0

BASKIN-ROBBINS

	AMOUNT	CALORIES	FAT-GRAMS	% FAT

BOSTON MARKET

BAKED GOODS

	AMOUNT	CALORIES	FAT-GRAMS	% FAT
Brownie	1	450	27	53
Chocolate Chip Cookie	1	340	17	45
Corn Bread	1 loaf	200	6	27
Oatmeal Raisin Cookie	1	320	13	37
Honey Wheat Roll	1	110	3	25

COLD SIDE DISHES

	AMOUNT	CALORIES	FAT-GRAMS	% FAT
Caesar Salad	1 serving	210	17	73
Coleslaw	1 serving	280	16	51
Cranberry Relish	1 serving	370	5	12
Fruit Salad	1 serving	70	0	0
Mediterranean Pasta Salad	1 serving	170	10	53
Tortellini Salad	1 serving	380	24	57

ENTRÉES

	AMOUNT	CALORIES	FAT-GRAMS	% FAT
Chicken Pot Pie	1 serving	750	34	41
¼ Chicken, white meat				
w/o Skin & Wing	1 serving	160	4	22
w/ Skin	1 serving	330	17	46
¼ Chicken, dark meat				
w/o Skin	1 serving	210	10	43
w/ Skin	1 serving	330	22	59
½ Chicken, w/ Skin	1 serving	630	37	53
Chicken Salad, Chunky	1 serving	370	27	66
Ham w/ Cinnamon				
Apples	1 serving	350	13	33
Meat Loaf & Chunky				
Tomato Sauce	1 serving	370	18	44

	AMOUNT	CALORIES	FAT-GRAMS	% FAT
Meat Loaf & Brown Gravy	l serving	390	22	51
Turkey Breast, Skinless Rotisserie	l serving	170	1	5

HOT SIDE DISHES

BBQ Baked Beans	l serving	330	9	25
Chicken Gravy	l oz	15	9	60
Corn, Whole Kernel	l serving	180	4	20
Green Bean Casserole	l serving	90	5	50
Hot Cinnamon Apples	l serving	250	5	18
Macaroni and Cheese	l serving	280	10	32
Potatoes, Mashed	l serving	180	8	40
& Gravy	l serving	200	9	41
Potatoes, New	l serving	130	3	20
Rice Pilaf	l serving	180	5	25
Spinach, Creamed	l serving	280	21	68
Squash, Butternut	l serving	160	6	34
Stuffing	l serving	310	12	35
Vegetables, Steamed	l serving	35	.5	13
Zucchini Marinara	l serving	80	4	44

SOUPS, SALADS & SANDWICHES

Soups

Chicken	l serving	80	3	34
Chicken Tortilla	l serving	220	11	45

	AMOUNT	CALORIES	FAT-GRAMS	% FAT
Salads				
Caesar, Entrée	1 serving	520	43	74
w/o Dressing	1 serving	240	13	49
Chicken Caesar	1 serving	670	47	63
Sandwiches				
Chicken	1	430	5	10
Chicken w/ Cheese				
& Sauce	1	750	33	40
Chicken Salad	1	680	30	40
Ham	1	450	9	18
Ham w/ Cheese & Sauce	1	760	35	41
Ham & Turkey Club	1	430	6	13
Ham & Turkey Club				
w/ Cheese & Sauce	1	890	44	44
Meat Loaf	1	690	21	27
w/ Cheese & Sauce	1	860	33	35
Turkey	1	400	4	9
Turkey w/ Cheese &				
Sauce	1	710	28	35

BURGER KING

BREAKFAST ITEMS

	AMOUNT	CALORIES	FAT-GRAMS	% FAT
Bagel				
Plain	1	270	6	20
w/ Cream Cheese	1	370	16	39
w/ Bacon, Egg &				
Cheese	1	455	20	40
w/ Egg & Cheese	1	410	16	35

	AMOUNT	CALORIES	FAT-GRAMS	% FAT
w/ Ham, Egg & Cheese	1	440	17	35
w/ Sausage, Egg & Cheese	1	625	36	52
Biscuit				
Plain	1	330	17	46
w/ Bacon	1	380	20	48
w/ Bacon & Egg	1	470	27	52
w/ Sausage	1	590	40	61
w/ Sausage & Egg	1	570	36	52
Breakfast Buddy	1	255	16	56
Croissant, Plain	1	180	10	50
Croissan'wich				
w/ Bacon, Egg & Cheese	1	510	31	55
w/ Sausage, Egg & Cheese	1	600	46	69
Danish				
Apple Cinnamon	1	390	13	30
Cheese	1	405	16	35
Cinnamon Raisin	1	450	18	36
French Toast Sticks	1 order	500	27	49
Mini Muffins				
Blueberry	1	290	14	43
Lemon Poppyseed	1	320	18	51
Raisin Oat Bran	1	290	12	37
Scrambled Egg Platter				
Regular	1	550	34	56
w/ Bacon	1	610	39	58
w/ Sausage	1	770	53	62

BURGER KING

	AMOUNT	CALORIES	FAT-GRAMS	% FAT

CHEESEBURGERS & HAMBURGERS

Cheeseburgers

Big King	1	600	36	54
Deluxe	1	390	23	53
Double	1	600	36	54
w/ Bacon	1	640	39	55
Double Whopper w/ Cheese	1	960	63	59
Regular	1	380	19	45
Whopper w/ Cheese	1	730	46	57
Whopper Jr. w/ Cheese	1	460	28	55

Hamburgers

Double Whopper	1	870	56	58
Regular	1	330	15	41
Whopper	1	640	39	55
Whopper Jr.	1	410	24	53

CHICKEN

Chicken Tenders	6 pcs	230	12	47

DESSERT

Dutch Apple Pie	1 serving	300	15	45

DRINKS & SHAKES

Drinks

Coca-Cola, Medium	1	260	0	0
Diet Coke, Medium	1	0	0	0
Milk				
2%	1 serving	120	5	37
Whole	1 serving	160	9	52

	AMOUNT	CALORIES	FAT-GRAMS	% FAT
Orange Juice	I serving	160	0	0
Sprite, Medium	I	260	0	0
Shakes				
Chocolate, Medium	I	320	7	20
w/ Syrup Added	I	440	7	14
Strawberry, Medium, w/ Syrup Added	I	420	6	13
Vanilla, Medium	I	300	6	18

ONIONS & POTATOES

Onions

	AMOUNT	CALORIES	FAT-GRAMS	% FAT
Onion Rings	I serving	310	14	41
Potatoes				
French Fries	I reg serving	230	13	52
	I med serving	370	20	49
Hash Browns	I serving	220	12	49

SALADS & SALAD DRESSINGS

Salads

	AMOUNT	CALORIES	FAT-GRAMS	% FAT
Broiled Chicken	I serving	200	10	45
Chef	I serving	180	9	46
Chunky Chicken	I serving	140	4	25
Garden	I serving	100	5	45
Side	I serving	60	3	45

BURGER KING

	AMOUNT	CALORIES	FAT-GRAMS	% FAT
Salad Dressings				
Bleu Cheese	1 pkt	300	32	96
French	1 pkt	290	22	68
House	1 pkt	260	26	35
Light Italian	1 pkt	170	18	95
Olive Oil &				
Vinegar	1 pkt	310	33	96
Ranch	1 pkt	350	37	95
Thousand Island	1 pkt	290	26	81
SANDWICHES				
Chicken				
BK Broiler	1	550	29	47
Fried Chicken	1	710	43	55
Fish				
BK Big Fish	1	700	41	53
SAUCES				
BK Broiler Sauce	½ oz	90	10	100
Burger King				
AM Express	1 oz	85	0	0
Dipping Sauces				
Barbecue	1 oz	35	0	0
Honey	1 oz	90	0	0
Ranch	1 oz	170	18	95
Sweet & Sour	1 oz	45	0	0
Mayonnaise	1 oz	195	21	97
Mustard	1 pkt	5	0	0
Tartar Sauce	1 oz	135	14	94

CARL'S JR.

	AMOUNT	CALORIES	FAT-GRAMS	% FAT
BREAKFAST ITEMS				
Bacon	2 strips	50	4	72
Cinnamon Roll	1	460	18	35
Danish Pastry				
All types except				
cheese	1	520	16	28
Cheese	1	520	22	38
English Muffin				
w/ Margarine	1	180	6	30
French Toast Dips,				
w/o Syrup	1 serving	480	26	48
Hot Cakes,				
w/ Margarine,				
w/o Syrup	1 serving	360	12	30
Muffins				
Blueberry	1	340	9	24
Bran	1	310	7	20
Sausage Patty	1 serving	190	17	81
Scrambled Eggs	1 serving	120	9	68
Sunrise Sandwich	1	300	13	39
w/ Bacon	1	370	19	46
w/ Sausage	1	500	32	58
CHEESEBURGERS				
& HAMBURGERS				
Cheeseburgers				
Double Western				
Bacon	1	1,030	63	55
Western Bacon	1	730	39	48

	AMOUNT	CALORIES	FAT-GRAMS	% FAT
Hamburgers				
Big Burger	1	470	20	38
Carl's Original	1	460	20	39
Famous Star	1	610	38	56
Happy Star	1	200	8	36
Old Time Star	1	400	17	38
Regular	1	320	14	39
Super Star	1	820	53	58
CHICKEN				
Chicken Stars	6 pcs	230	14	55
Chicken Strips	6 pcs	260	19	66
DESSERTS				
Cake				
Chocolate	1 serving	300	11	33
Fudge Mousecake	1 serving	400	23	52
Cheesecake	1 serving	310	17	49
Chocolate Chip				
Cookie	1	330	17	46
Fudge Brownie	1	597	27	41
DRINKS & SHAKES				
Drinks				
Carbonated Drink,				
Medium	1	240	0	0
Diet	1	0	0	0
Iced Tea	20 oz	0	0	0
Milk, 1%	10 oz	150	3	18
Orange Juice, Small	1	90	1	18

	AMOUNT	CALORIES	FAT-GRAMS	% FAT
Shakes (All Flavors)				
Small	1	270	5	17
Regular	1	350	7	18
Large	1	460	9	18
HOT DOGS				
All Star	1	540	35	58
Chili Dog	1	720	47	59
ONIONS & POTATOES				
Onions				
Onion Rings				
Large	1 serving	520	26	45
Medium	1 serving	310	15	44
Potatoes				
Baked				
Bacon & Cheese	1	730	43	53
Broccoli & Cheese	1	590	31	47
Cheese	1	690	36	47
Fiesta	1	720	38	48
Lite	1	290	1	3
Sour Cream &				
Chive	1	470	19	36
French Fries				
Small	1 serving	280	13	42
Regular	1 serving	420	20	43
Large	1 serving	545	26	43
Criss-Cut	1 serving	330	22	60
Hash Brown Nuggets	1 serving	270	17	57

CARL'S JR.

	AMOUNT	CALORIES	FAT-GRAMS	% FAT
SALADS & SALAD DRESSINGS				
Salads				
Charbroiled				
Chicken	1	260	9	31
Chefs	1	180	7	35
Chicken	1	200	8	36
Garden	1	50	3	54
Garden, Lite	1	50	3	54
Lite Chicken	1	200	8	36
Teriyaki	1	330	6	16
Taco	1	355	19	48
Salad Dressings				
Bleu Cheese	1 oz	150	15	90
French, Reduced-Cal	1 oz	40	2	45
House	1 oz	110	11	90
Italian	1 oz	120	13	98
Italian, Reduced-Cal	1 oz	40	2	45
Thousand Island	1 oz	110	11	90
SANDWICHES				
Chicken				
Bacon Swiss	1	670	36	48
Charbroiler BBQ	1	310	6	17
Charbroiler Club	1	570	29	46
Sante Fe	1	530	29	49
Teriyaki Lite	1	330	6	16
Fish				
Carl's Catch	1	560	30	48
Fillet	1	550	26	43

	AMOUNT	CALORIES	FAT-GRAMS	% FAT
Roast Beef				
California Roast Beef				
'n Swiss	1	360	8	20
Club	1	620	34	49
Deluxe	1	540	26	43
Steak, Country Fried	1	610	33	49
Turkey, Club	1	530	23	39
SAUCES				
Guacamole	1 pkt	50	4	72
Salsa	1 pkt	10	0	0
Taco Sauce	1 pkt	10	0	0
SOUPS				
Boston Clam				
Chowder	1 serving	140	8	51
Chicken Noodle	1 serving	80	1	11
Cream of Broccoli	1 serving	140	6	39
Vegetable	1 serving	70	3	39

CHURCH'S FRIED CHICKEN

CHICKEN, FILLET

	AMOUNT	CALORIES	FAT-GRAMS	% FAT
Breast	1 serving	610	34	50
w/ Cheese	1 serving	250	16	58

CHICKEN, FRIED

	AMOUNT	CALORIES	FAT-GRAMS	% FAT
Breast				
Boneless	1 serving	200	12	56
Fried	1 serving	280	17	55

	AMOUNT	CALORIES	FAT-GRAMS	% FAT
& Wing, Fried	1 serving	305	20	55
w/ Corn	1 serving	280	16	42
Leg				
Fried	1 serving	150	9	53
Boneless	1 serving	140	9	59
w/ Cajun Rice	1 serving	270	16	53
Thigh				
Fried	1 serving	305	22	65
Boneless	1 serving	230	16	63
2 Thighs w/				
Biscuit	1 serving	710	49	62
Wing				
Boneless	1 serving	250	16	58
2 Wings w/ Biscuit	1 serving	750	49	59
Nuggets	6 pieces	330	19	51
DESSERTS				
Apple Pie	1 serving	280	12	40
Frozen Dessert	1 serving	180	6	30
Pecan Pie	1 serving	370	20	48
FISH FILLETS				
Regular	1 serving	430	18	38
w/ Cheese	1 serving	485	22	41
Fried Catfish	3 pieces	200	12	54
HOT DOGS				
Regular				
w/ Cheese	1	330	21	57
w/ Chili	1	320	20	56

	AMOUNT	CALORIES	FAT-GRAMS	% FAT
Super	1	520	27	47
w/ Cheese	1	580	34	53
w/ Chili	1	570	32	51

OTHER ITEMS

	AMOUNT	CALORIES	FAT-GRAMS	% FAT
Biscuit	1	250	16	59
Coleslaw	1 serving	90	6	54
Corn on the Cob	1	190	5	26
w/ Butter oil	1	240	9	34
Dinner Roll	1	85	2	17
French Fries				
Regular	1 serving	210	11	45
Large	1 serving	320	16	45
Hush Puppy	2 pieces	160	6	35
Okra	1 serving	210	16	69
Onion Rings	1 serving	280	16	51
Potatoes, Mashed,				
w/ Gravy	1 serving	90	3	33
Rice, Cajun	1 serving	130	7	48

DAIRY QUEEN/BRAZIER

CHEESEBURGERS & HAMBURGERS

Cheeseburgers

	AMOUNT	CALORIES	FAT-GRAMS	% FAT
Bacon Double	1	610	36	53
Deluxe Double	1	540	31	52
Double	1	540	31	52
Regular	1	340	17	45

	AMOUNT	CALORIES	FAT-GRAMS	% FAT
Hamburgers				
Double	1	440	22	45
Regular	1	290	12	37
Ultimate	1	670	43	58
CHICKEN				
Chicken Strip Basket				
w/ Gravy	1 serving	860	42	44
w/ BBQ Sauce	1 serving	810	37	41
DESSERTS				
Hot Fudge Brownie				
Delight	1 serving	710	29	37
Cake				
Frozen,				
Undecorated	1 serving	380	18	43
Strawberry				
Shortcake	1 serving	540	11	18
DESSERTS, FROZEN				
Banana Split	1	510	11	19
Blizzard				
Butterfinger				
Small	1	520	18	31
Regular	1	750	26	31
Chocolate Chip Cookie				
Dough				
Small	1	660	24	33
Regular	1	950	36	34

	AMOUNT	CALORIES	FAT-GRAMS	% FAT
Chocolate Sandwich Cookie				
Small	1	520	18	31
Regular	1	640	23	32
Health				
Small	1	560	23	37
Regular	1	820	36	40
Reese's Peanut Butter Cup				
Small	1	590	24	36
Regular	1	790	33	38
Strawberry				
Small	1	400	11	25
Regular	1	570	16	25
Breeze				
Heath				
Small	1	470	10	19
Regular	1	710	18	23
Strawberry				
Small	1	320	.5	1
Regular	1	460	1	2
Bars				
Buster Bar	1	450	28	56
Caramel & Nut Bar	1	260	13	45
Chocolate Dilly Bar	1	210	13	56
Chocolate Mint Dilly Bar	1	190	12	57
Fudge Bar	1	50	0	0
Fudge Nut Bar	1	410	25	55
Toffee Dilly Bar	1	210	12	51
Vanilla Orange Bar	1	60	0	0

	AMOUNT	CALORIES	FAT-GRAMS	% FAT
Chipper Sandwich	1	320	7	20
Cone, Ice Cream				
Chocolate				
Small	1	240	8	30
Regular	1	360	11	28
Vanilla				
Small	1	230	7	27
Regular	1	350	10	26
Large	1	410	12	26
Cone, Soft Serve, Dipped				
Small	1	340	17	45
Regular	1	510	25	44
Cone, Yogurt	1	280	1	3
Double Delight	1	490	20	37
DQ Sandwich	1	150	5	30
Frozen Log Cake	⅛ of cake	280	9	29
Frozen Heart Cake	⅒ of cake	270	9	30
Frozen 8" Round Cake	⅛ of cake	340	12	32
Frozen 10" Round Cake	⅟₁₂ of cake	360	12	30
Frozen Sheet Cake	⅟₂₀ of cake	350	12	31
Parfait, Peanut Butter	1	730	31	38
Queens Choice				
Big Scoop				
Chocolate	1	250	14	50
Vanilla	1	250	14	50
Soft Serve				
Chocolate	½ cup	150	5	30
Vanilla	½ cup	140	4.5	29

	AMOUNT	CALORIES	FAT-GRAMS	% FAT
Sundae				
Chocolate				
Small	1	290	7	22
Regular	1	410	10	22
Strawberry Yogurt	1	300	.5	2
Strawberry Waffle Cone	1	350	12	31
Treatzza Pizza				
Heath	⅛ of pizza	180	7	35
M&M	⅛ of pizza	190	7	33
Strawberry-Banana	⅛ of pizza	180	6	30
Peanut Butter Fudge	⅛ of pizza	220	10	41
Yogurt, Nonfat Frozen	½ cup	100	0	0
DRINKS, MALTS & SHAKES				
Drinks				
Cooler, Strawberry	1	190	0	0
Float	1	410	7	15
Freeze	1	500	12	22
Slush				
Small	1	220	0	0
Regular	1	290	0	0
Malts				
Chocolate				
Small	1	650	16	22
Regular	1	880	22	23
Shakes				
Chocolate				
Small	1	560	15	24
Regular	1	770	20	23

	AMOUNT	CALORIES	FAT-GRAMS	% FAT
HOT DOGS				
Cheese Dog	1	290	18	56
Chili Dog	1	280	16	51
Chili 'n' Cheese Dog	1	330	21	57
Regular	1	240	14	53
ONIONS & POTATOES				
Onions				
Onion Rings	1 serving	240	12	45
Potatoes				
French Fries				
Small	1 serving	210	10	43
Regular	1 serving	300	14	42
Large	1 serving	390	18	42
SALADS & SALAD DRESSINGS				
Salads				
Garden, w/o Dressing	1 serving	200	13	59
Side, w/o Dressing	1 serving	25	0	0
Salad Dressings				
French, Reduced-Calorie	1 serving	90	5	50
Thousand Island	1 serving	225	21	84
SANDWICHES				
BBQ Beef	1	225	4	16
Chicken Breast Fillet	1	430	20	42
w/ Cheese	1	480	25	47

	AMOUNT	CALORIES	FAT-GRAMS	% FAT
Fish Fillet	1	370	16	39
w/ Cheese	1	420	21	45

DEL TACO

	AMOUNT	CALORIES	FAT-GRAMS	% FAT
Burritos				
Beef	1	440	20	41
"Big Del"	1	455	20	40
Breakfast	1	255	11	39
Chicken	1	265	10	34
Chicken Fajita, Deluxe	1	435	22	46
Combination	1	415	17	37
Green	1	230	8	31
Large	1	330	11	30
Macho Combo	1	775	31	36
Red	1	235	8	31
Large	1	340	11	29
Cheeseburger	1	340	11	29
Chicken Salad	1 serving	255	19	67
French Fries	1 serving	240	11	41
Guacamole	2 tbsp	60	6	90
Hamburger	1	230	8	31
Quesadilla, Regular	1	485	27	50
Refried Beans				
w/ Cheese	1 serving	120	7	52
Salsa	4 tbsp	15	0	0
Taco				
Chicken Fajita, Deluxe	1	210	10	43
Double Beef, Deluxe, Soft	1	210	11	47

DEL TACO

	AMOUNT	CALORIES	FAT-GRAMS	% FAT
Soft				
Small	1	145	6	37
Regular	1	210	10	43
Tostado	1	140	8	51

D'LITES OF AMERICA

CHEESEBURGERS & HAMBURGERS

Cheeseburgers

Cheeseburger w/ Bacon

	AMOUNT	CALORIES	FAT-GRAMS	% FAT
on multi-grain bun	1	370	18	44
on sesame seed bun	1	280	18	44

Hamburgers

	AMOUNT	CALORIES	FAT-GRAMS	% FAT
Jr. D'Lite	1	200	7	32
¼ lb D'Lite	1	280	12	39
Double D'Lite	1	450	22	44

DESSERT

	AMOUNT	CALORIES	FAT-GRAMS	% FAT
Chocolate D'Lite	1	205	4	18

POTATOES

Baked

	AMOUNT	CALORIES	FAT-GRAMS	% FAT
Mexican	1	510	18	32
Regular	1	230	1	4
w/ Bacon & Cheddar Cheese	1	490	20	37
w/ Broccoli & Cheddar Cheese	1	410	16	35

	AMOUNT	CALORIES	FAT-GRAMS	% FAT
French Fries				
Regular	1 serving	260	12	42
Large	1 serving	320	15	42
Skins				
Mexi Skins	1 serving	100	7	64
Regular	1 serving	90	6	60

SALAD & SALAD DRESSING

Salad

	AMOUNT	CALORIES	FAT-GRAMS	% FAT
Salad Bar Platter	1 serving	130	6	42

Salad Dressing

	AMOUNT	CALORIES	FAT-GRAMS	% FAT
Mayonnaise, Lite	1 tbsp	40	4	90

SANDWICHES

	AMOUNT	CALORIES	FAT-GRAMS	% FAT
Chicken Fillet	1	280	11	35
Fish Fillet	1	390	21	48
Tartar Sauce, Lite	1 tbsp	60	6	90
Ham & Cheese	1	280	8	26
Vegetarian	1	270	14	47

DOMINO'S PIZZA

12" MEDIUM CHEESE PIZZAS

	AMOUNT	CALORIES	FAT-GRAMS	% FAT
Hand-Tossed	2 of 8 slices	350	11	28
Thin Crust	¼ of pizza	275	12	39
Deep Dish	2 of 8 slices	465	21	41

	AMOUNT	CALORIES	FAT-GRAMS	% FAT
For toppings, add the following:				
Anchovies	avg portion	20	1	45
Bacon	avg portion	80	7	79
Banana Peppers	avg portion	5	0	0
Beef, Precooked	avg portion	55	5	82
Cheese				
Cheddar	avg portion	60	5	75
Extra	avg portion	50	4	72
Green Peppers	avg portion	5	0	0
Ham	avg portion	20	1	45
Italian Sausage	avg portion	55	5	82
Mushrooms, Canned	avg portion	5	0	0
Fresh	avg portion	5	0	0
Olives				
Green	avg portion	15	1	60
Ripe	avg portion	15	1	60

	AMOUNT	CALORIES	FAT-GRAMS	% FAT
Onion	avg portion	5	0	0
Pepperoni	avg portion	60	5	75
Pineapple Tidbits	avg portion	10	0	0

14" LARGE CHEESE PIZZAS

	AMOUNT	CALORIES	FAT-GRAMS	% FAT
Hand-Tossed	2 of 12 slices	320	10	28
Thin Crust	⅙ of pizza	255	11	39
Deep Dish	2 of 12 slices	465	20	39

For toppings, add the following:

	AMOUNT	CALORIES	FAT-GRAMS	% FAT
Anchovies	avg portion	20	1	45
Bacon	avg portion	75	6	72
Banana Peppers	avg portion	5	0	0
Beef, Precooked	avg portion	45	4	80
Cheese Cheddar	avg portion	50	4	72
Extra	avg portion	45	4	80
Green Peppers	avg portion	5	0	0

	AMOUNT	CALORIES	FAT-GRAMS	% FAT
Ham	avg			
	portion	15	1	60
Italian Sausage	avg			
	portion	45	4	80
Mushrooms				
Canned	avg			
	portion	5	0	0
Fresh	avg			
	portion	5	0	0
Olives				
Green	avg			
	portion	10	1	90
Ripe	avg			
	portion	10	1	90
Onion	avg			
	portion	5	0	0
Pepperoni	avg			
	portion	55	5	82
Pineapple Tidbits	avg			
	portion	10	0	0

6" DEEP-DISH CHEESE PIZZAS

	AMOUNT	CALORIES	FAT-GRAMS	% FAT
Cheese Pizza	1 pizza	590	27	41

For toppings, add the following:

	AMOUNT	CALORIES	FAT-GRAMS	% FAT
Anchovies	avg			
	portion	45	2	40
Bacon	avg			
	portion	80	7	79

	AMOUNT	CALORIES	FAT-GRAMS	% FAT
Banana Peppers	avg portion	5	0	0
Beef, Precooked	avg portion	55	5	82
Cheese Cheddar	avg portion	85	7	74
Extra	avg portion	50	4	72
Green Peppers	avg portion	5	0	0
Ham	avg portion	15	1	60
Italian Sausage	avg portion	45	4	80
Mushrooms Canned	avg portion	5	0	0
Fresh	avg portion	5	0	0
Olives Green	avg portion	10	1	90
Ripe	avg portion	10	1	90
Onion	avg portion	5	0	0
Pepperoni	avg portion	50	5	90

	AMOUNT	CALORIES	FAT-GRAMS	% FAT
Pineapple Tidbits	avg portion	10	0	0

OTHER FOODS

Buffalo Wings

	AMOUNT	CALORIES	FAT-GRAMS	% FAT
Barbeque	1 wing	50	3	54
Hot	1 wing	45	3	60

Bread

Bread Sticks	1 pc	80	4	45
Cheesy Bread	1 pc	105	6	51

Salad

Garden

Small	1	20	0	0
Large	1	40	0	0

Salad Dressings

Creamy Caesar	1 serving	200	22	99
Blue Cheese	1 serving	220	24	98
Honey French	1 serving	210	18	77

Italian

House	1 serving	220	24	98
Light	1 serving	20	1	45

Ranch

Fat-Free	1 serving	40	0	0
Regular	1 serving	260	29	100
Thousand Island	1 serving	200	20	90

	AMOUNT	CALORIES	FAT-GRAMS	% FAT
DUNKIN' DONUTS				
BAGELS				
Cinnamon 'N Raisin	1	250	2	7
Egg	1	250	2	7
Onion	1	230	1	4
Plain	1	240	1	4
COOKIES				
Chocolate Chunk	1	200	10	45
w/ Nuts	1	210	11	47
Oatmeal Pecan Raisin	1	200	9	41
CROISSANTS				
Almond	1	420	27	58
Chocolate	1	440	29	59
Plain	1	310	19	55
DONUTS				
Apple-Filled Cinnamon	1	250	11	40
Bavarian-Filled				
w/ Chocolate Frosting	1	240	11	41
Blueberry-Filled	1	210	8	34
"Boston Kreme"	1	240	11	41
Cinnamon,				
Apple-Filled	1	190	9	43
Chocolate Frosted				
Yeast Ring	1	200	10	45
Cruller				
Glazed French	1	140	8	51
Honey-Dipped	1	260	11	38

	AMOUNT	CALORIES	FAT-GRAMS	% FAT
Glazed				
Buttermilk	1	290	14	43
Chocolate	1	325	21	58
Coffee Roll	1	280	12	39
Whole Wheat	1	330	18	49
Yeast Ring	1	200	9	41
Jelly-Filled Donut	1	220	9	37
Lemon-Filled Donut	1	260	12	42
Plain				
Cake	1	270	17	57
Cake, w/ Handle	1	240	14	53
Powdered, Cake	1	270	16	53
MUFFINS				
Apple 'N Spice	1	300	8	24
Banana Nut	1	310	10	29
Blueberry	1	280	8	26
Bran w/ Raisins	1	310	9	26
Corn	1	240	12	32
Cranberry Nut	1	290	9	28
Oat Bran	1	330	11	30

EL POLLO LOCO

BURRITOS				
Bean, Rice, Cheese	1	530	13	22
Chicken	1	310	11	32
Classic	1	560	20	32
Loco Grande	1	680	30	40
Spicy Hot	1	570	20	32

	AMOUNT	CALORIES	FAT-GRAMS	% FAT
Whole Wheat	1	510	16	28
Steak	1	450	22	44
Grilled	1	740	29	35
Vegetarian	1	340	7	19

CHICKEN

Breast	1	160	6	34
Leg	1	90	5	50
Thigh	1	180	12	60
Wing	1	110	6	49

DESSERTS

"Orange Bang"	1 serving	110	0	0
"Piña Colada Bang"	1 serving	110	0	0

FAJITA ENTRÉE
w/ Rice, Beans,
   3 Tortillas, Salsa

Chicken	1 serving	780	18	21
Steak	1 serving	1,040	38	33

SALADS & SALAD DRESSINGS
Salads

Chicken	1 serving	160	4	23
Potato	1 serving	180	10	50
Side	1 serving	50	1	18

Salad Dressings

Blue Cheese	1 oz	80	6	68
French "DeLuxe"	1 oz	60	4	80

	AMOUNT	CALORIES	FAT-GRAMS	% FAT
Italian,				
Reduced-Cal	1 oz	25	2	72
Ranch	1 oz	75	6	72
Thousand Island	1 oz	110	10	82
TACOS				
Chicken	1	180	7	35
Steak	1	250	12	43
OTHER ITEMS				
Beans	1 serving	100	3	27
Coleslaw	1 serving	90	8	80
Corn	1 serving	110	2	16
Guacamole	1 oz	60	6	90
Rice	1 serving	110	2	16
Salsa	2 oz	10	0	0
Sour Cream	1 oz	60	6	90
Tortilla				
Corn	1	60	1	8
Flour	1	90	3	30

GODFATHER'S PIZZA

ORIGINAL CRUST

Cheese Pizza

	AMOUNT	CALORIES	FAT-GRAMS	% FAT
Mini	¼ pie	130	3	21
Medium	⅛ pie	230	5	20
Large	⅒ pie	260	6	21
Jumbo	⅒ pie	380	9	21

	AMOUNT	CALORIES	FAT-GRAMS	% FAT
Combo Pizza				
Mini	¼ pie	175	7	36
Medium	⅛ pie	305	11	32
Large	⅒ pie	340	12	32
Jumbo	⅒ pie	505	18	32
GOLDEN CRUST				
Cheese Pizza				
Medium	⅛ pie	210	8	34
Large	⅒ pie	240	9	34
Combo Pizza				
Medium	⅛ pie	370	12	29
Large	⅒ pie	305	12	41

HARDEE'S

BREAKFAST ITEMS				
Big Country Breakfast				
w/ Bacon	1 serving	820	49	53
w/ Sausage	1 serving	1,000	66	59
Biscuits				
Bacon & Egg	1	570	33	52
Bacon, Egg & Cheese	1	610	37	54
Apple Cinnamon				
'N' Raisin	1	200	8	36
Country Ham	1	430	22	46
Ham	1	400	20	45
Ham, Egg & Cheese	1	540	30	50

	AMOUNT	CALORIES	FAT-GRAMS	% FAT
Jelly Biscuit	1	440	21	43
'N Gravy	1	510	28	49
Rise 'N' Shine	1	390	21	48
Sausage	1	510	31	55
Sausage & Egg	1	630	40	57
Ultimate Omelet	1	570	33	52
Fried Egg	1	80	6	74
Frisco Breakfast				
Sandwich (Ham)	1	500	25	45
Hash Rounds	1	230	14	55
Pancakes	3	280	2	6
w/ 1 Sausage Patty	3	430	16	33
w/ 2 Bacon Strips	3	350	9	23

CHEESEBURGERS & HAMBURGERS

Cheeseburgers

	AMOUNT	CALORIES	FAT-GRAMS	% FAT
Cravin' Bacon	1	690	46	60
Mesquite Bacon	1	370	18	44
Mushroom				
'N' Swiss	1	490	25	46
Quarter-Pound				
Double	1	470	27	52
Regular	1	310	14	41

Hamburgers

	AMOUNT	CALORIES	FAT-GRAMS	% FAT
Frisco Burger	1	720	46	58
Regular	1	270	11	37
The Boss	1	570	33	52
The Works	1	530	30	51

	AMOUNT	CALORIES	FAT-GRAMS	% FAT
CHICKEN, FRIED				
Breast	1 serving	370	15	36
Leg	1 serving	170	7	37
Stix	6 pcs	210	9	39
	9 pcs	310	14	41
Thigh	1 serving	330	15	41
Wing	1 serving	200	8	36
DESSERTS				
Apple Turnover	1	270	12	40
Big Cookie	1	280	12	39
Cone				
Chocolate	1	180	2	10
Vanilla	1	170	2	11
Cool Twist Cone				
Vanilla/Chocolate	1	120	2	10
Cool Twist Sundae				
Hot Fudge	1	290	6	18
Strawberry	1	210	2	8
Peach Cobbler	1 serving, small	310	7	20
DRINKS & SHAKES				
Milk, 2%	1	120	4	33
Orange Juice	1	140	0	0
Shakes				
Chocolate	1	370	5	12
Peach	1	390	4	9
Strawberry	1	420	4	9
Vanilla	1	350	5	12

HARDEE'S

	AMOUNT	CALORIES	FAT-GRAMS	% FAT
POTATOES				
French Fries				
Small	1 serving	240	10	38
Medium	1 serving	350	15	39
Large	1 serving	430	18	38
Hash Rounds	1 serving	230	14	55
Mashed	1 serving	70	1	12
SALADS & SALAD DRESSINGS				
Salads				
Chicken, Grilled	1	150	3	18
Garden	1	220	13	53
Side	1	25	0	0
Salad Dressings				
French, Fat-Free	1 pkt	70	0	0
French, Reduced-Calorie	1 pkt	130	5	35
House	1 pkt	290	29	90
Italian, Reduced-Calorie	1 pkt	90	8	80
Ranch	1 pkt	290	29	90
Thousand Island	1 pkt	250	23	83
SANDWICHES				
Chicken Fillet	1	480	18	34
Chicken, Grilled	1	350	11	28
Fisherman's Fillet	1	560	27	43
Hot Ham 'N' Cheese	1	310	12	35
Roast Beef, Regular	1	320	16	45
Roast Beef, Big	1	460	24	47

	AMOUNT	CALORIES	FAT-GRAMS	% FAT
OTHER ITEMS				
Baked Beans	I serving, small	170	I	<I
Barbecue Sauce	I pkt	15	0	0
Coleslaw, Small	I serving	240	20	75
Coleslaw, Large	I serving	710	60	76
Dipping Sauces				
BBQ	I pkt	30	0	0
Big Twin	I pkt	50	4	72
Honey	I pkt	45	0	0
Sweet Mustard	I pkt	50	0	0
Sweet 'n' Sour	I pkt	40	0	0
Gravy, 1.5 oz	I serving	20	tr	2
Gravy, 5 oz	I serving	60	I	5
Horseradish	I serving	25	2	75
Mayonnaise	I serving	50	5	90
Syrup, Pancake	I serving	120	0	0
Tartar Sauce	I serving	90	9	90

JACK IN THE BOX

BREAKFAST ITEMS

	AMOUNT	CALORIES	FAT-GRAMS	% FAT
Sandwich				
Breakfast Jack	I	300	12	36
Sourdough	I	380	21	50
Ultimate	I	620	36	521
Croissant				
Sausage	I	670	48	64
Supreme	I	570	20	32
Pancakes w/ Bacon	I serving	160	12	68

	AMOUNT	CALORIES	FAT-GRAMS	% FAT
CHEESEBURGERS & HAMBURGERS				
Cheeseburgers				
Bacon Ultimate	1	1,150	89	70
Double	1	450	24	48
Jumbo Jack	1	650	43	60
Regular	1	330	15	41
Ultimate	1	1,030	79	69
Hamburgers				
Jumbo Jack	1	560	36	58
Quarter Pound	1	510	27	48
Regular	1	280	12	39
DESSERTS				
Cheesecake	1 serving	310	18	51
Carrot Cake	1 serving	370	16	39
Double Fudge Cake	1 serving	300	10	30
Hot Apple Turnover	1	340	18	48
DRINKS & SHAKES				
Drinks (Regular Size)				
Coffee	1	5	0	0
Iced Tea	1	0	0	0
Lemonade	1	190	0	0
Milk, 2%	1	130	5	35
Orange Juice	1	150	0	0
Soft Drinks,				
Coca-Cola Classic	1	170	0	0
Barq's Root Beer	1	180	0	0

	AMOUNT	CALORIES	FAT-GRAMS	% FAT
Diet Coke	I	0	0	0
Dr Pepper	I	190	0	0
Sprite	I	160	0	0

Ice Cream Shakes (Regular Size)

	AMOUNT	CALORIES	FAT-GRAMS	% FAT
Cappuccino	I	630	29	41
Chocolate	I	610	31	46
Oreo Cookie	I	740	36	44
Strawberry	I	640	28	39
Vanilla	I	610	31	46

ONIONS & POTATOES

Onions

	AMOUNT	CALORIES	FAT-GRAMS	% FAT
Onion Rings	I serving	460	25	49

Potatoes

Curley Fries

	AMOUNT	CALORIES	FAT-GRAMS	% FAT
Chili Cheese	I serving	650	41	57
Seasoned	I serving	420	24	51

French Fries

	AMOUNT	CALORIES	FAT-GRAMS	% FAT
Regular	I serving	360	17	43
Jumbo	I serving	430	20	42
Super Scoop	I serving	610	28	41
Hash Browns	I serving	160	11	62
Wedges, Bacon & Cheddar	I serving	800	58	65

SALADS & SALAD DRESSINGS

Salads

	AMOUNT	CALORIES	FAT-GRAMS	% FAT
Garden Chicken	I	200	9	41

	AMOUNT	CALORIES	FAT-GRAMS	% FAT
Side	1	50	3	54
Salad Dressings				
Bleu Cheese	1 pkt	210	18	77
Buttermilk House	1 pkt	290	30	93
Italian, Low-Calorie	1 pkt	25	2	72
Thousand Island	1 pkt	250	24	86
SANDWICHES				
Chicken	1	450	26	52
Caesar	1	520	26	45
Fajita Pita	1	280	9	29
Grilled Fillet	1	520	26	40
Really Big	1	900	56	45
Spicy Crispy	1	560	27	43
Supreme	1	680	45	60
Philly Cheesesteak	1	520	25	43
OTHER ITEMS				
Chicken & Fries	1 serving	730	34	42
Chicken Breast Pieces (Breaded)	5 pcs	360	17	43
Chicken Teriyaki Bowl	1	670	4	5
Dipping Sauces				
Barbecue	1 pkt	45	0	0
Buttermilk House	1 pkt	130	13	90
Sweet & Sour	1 pkt	40	0	0
Tartar	1 pkt	150	15	61
Sour Cream	1 pkt	60	6	90

	AMOUNT	CALORIES	FAT-GRAMS	% FAT
Egg Roll	3 pcs	440	24	49
	5 pcs	730	41	51
Fish & Chips	1 serving	720	35	44
Stuffed Jalapeños	7 pcs	470	28	54
	10 pcs	680	40	53
Taco				
Regular	1	190	11	53
Monster	1	290	18	56
Syrup, Pancake	1.5 oz	120	0	0
Salsa	1 oz	10	0	0
Tortilla Chips	1 oz	140	6	39

KENNY ROGERS ROASTERS

CHICKEN

	AMOUNT	CALORIES	FAT-GRAMS	% FAT
¼ Chicken, White Meat				
w/ Skin	1 serving	245	11	39
w/o Skin & Wing*	1 serving	145	2	14
¼ Chicken, Dark Meat				
w/ Skin	1 serving	270	17	56
w/o Skin*	1 serving	170	7	39
½ Chicken				
w/ Skin	1 serving	515	28	48
w/o Skin*	1 serving	315	10	26

(skin removed by customer)*

	AMOUNT	CALORIES	FAT-GRAMS	% FAT
SANDWICHES				
BBQ Chicken Pita	1	400	7	16
Chicken Caesar Pita	1	605	35	53
Roasted Chicken Pita	1	685	35	47
Turkey	1	385	12	28
SALADS & SALAD DRESSINGS				
Salads				
Chicken Caesar*	1	285	9	27
Roasted Chicken*	1	290	10	30
Side Salad	1	25	0	0
Tomato Cucumber	1 serving	125	2	29

(* Skin removed by customer)

	AMOUNT	CALORIES	FAT-GRAMS	% FAT
Salad Dressings (2.5 oz)				
Blue Cheese	1 serving	370	39	95
Buttermilk Ranch	1 serving	430	48	100
Caesar	1 serving	340	36	95
Dijon Honey Mustard	1 serving	320	28	79
Fat-Free Italian	1 serving	35	0	0
Honey French	1 serving	350	29	75
Thousand Island	1 serving	330	33	90
OTHER ITEMS				
Chicken Noodle Soup	1 cup	55	1	18
	1 bowl	90	2	18
Chicken Pot Pie	1 serving	710	33	42
Cinnamon Apples	1 serving	200	5	23
Cole Slaw	1 serving	225	16	63

	AMOUNT	CALORIES	FAT-GRAMS	% FAT
Cornbread Stuffing	I serving	325	19	51
Corn Muffin	I	175	8	41
Corn on the Cob	I	70	1	11
Creamy Parmesan Spinach	I serving	120	6	39
Garlic Parsley Potatoes	I serving	260	12	42
Honey Baked Beans	I serving	150	2	13
Italian Green Beans	I serving	115	8	60
Macaroni & Cheese	I serving	200	6	26
Mashed Potatoes	I serving	295	14	43
Pasta Salad	I serving	235	6	12
w/ Sour Cream & Dill	I serving	235	16	61
Potato Salad	I serving	390	27	63
Rice Pilaf	I serving	175	5	24
Steamed Vegetables	I serving	50	0	0
Sweet Corn Niblets	I serving	110	0	0
Sweet Potato, Baked	I serving	265	0	0
Zucchini & Squash Santa Fe	I serving	70	5	54

KENTUCKY FRIED CHICKEN

CHICKEN
Original Recipe

	AMOUNT	CALORIES	FAT-GRAMS	% FAT
Breast	I serving	400	24	54
Drumstick	I serving	140	9	58
Thigh	I serving	250	18	65
Wing	I serving	140	10	64

	AMOUNT	CALORIES	FAT-GRAMS	% FAT
Extra Tasty Crispy				
Breast	I serving	470	28	54
Drumstick	I serving	190	II	52
Thigh	I serving	370	25	61
Wing	I serving	200	13	59
Hot & Spicy				
Breast	I serving	530	35	59
Drumstick	I serving	190	II	52
Thigh	I serving	370	27	66
Wing	I serving	210	15	64
Tender Roast/Honey BBQ				
Tender Roast				
Breast				
w/ Skin	I serving	250	II	40
w/o Skin	I serving	170	4	21
Drumstick				
w/ Skin	I serving	95	4	38
w/o Skin	I serving	65	2	28
Thigh				
w/ Skin	I serving	210	12	51
w/o Skin	I serving	105	5	43
Wing w/ Skin	I serving	120	8	60
CHICKEN SNACKS				
Crispy Strips				
Colonel's	3 pieces	260	16	55
Spicy Buffalo	3 pieces	350	19	49
Hot Wings	6 pieces	470	33	63

	AMOUNT	CALORIES	FAT-GRAMS	% FAT
POTATOES				
French Fries				
Regular	I serving	245	12	44
Crispy	I serving	210	11	47
Kentucky Fries	I serving	270	13	44
Mashed Potatoes				
Plain	I serving	60	0	0
w/ Gravy	I serving	120	6	45
Potato Salad	I serving	230	14	55
Potato Wedges	I serving	280	13	42
SALADS & SALAD DRESSINGS				
Salads				
Garden	I serving	15	0	0
Macaroni	I serving	250	17	62
Pasta	I serving	135	8	53
Vegetable Medley	I serving	125	4	29
Salad Dressings				
Italian	I oz	15	1	60
Ranch	I oz	170	18	95
SANDWICHES				
Original Recipe Chicken	I	495	22	40
BBQ Flavor Chicken	I	255	8	28
OTHER ITEMS				
Beans				
Barbecue Baked	I serving	190	3	14
Green	I serving	45	1	20

	AMOUNT	CALORIES	FAT-GRAMS	% FAT
Biscuit	1	180	10	50
Chicken Pot Pie	1 serving	770	42	49
Cole Slaw	1 serving	180	9	45
Corn on the Cob				
w/ Savory	1 serving	190	3	14
w/o Savory	1 serving	150	2	12
Corn Bread	1 serving	230	13	51
Macaroni &				
Cheese	1 serving	180	8	40
Mean Greens	1 serving	70	3	39
Sauce (per packet)				
Barbecue	1	35	1	15
Honey	1	50	0	0
Mustard	1	35	1	23
Sweet 'n Sour	1	60	1	9

LITTLE CAESAR'S PIZZA

PIZZA

	AMOUNT	CALORIES	FAT-GRAMS	% FAT
Baby Pan!Pan!	1 pie	525	22	38
Cheese				
Round, Pizza!Pizza!				
Small	1 pie	140	5	33
Medium	1 pie	155	5	29
Large	1 pie	170	6	32
Single Slice	1 serving	170	6	32
Square, Pizza!Pizza!				
Small	1 pie	185	6	29
Medium	1 pie	190	6	29
Large	1 pie	190	6	29

	AMOUNT	CALORIES	FAT-GRAMS	% FAT
Pepperoni, Combination, Single Slice	I serving	190	7	33

PIZZA ENTRÉE
	AMOUNT	CALORIES	FAT-GRAMS	% FAT
Cheese Pizza w/ Tossed Salad	I serving	600	21	32
Vegetable Pizza w/ Tossed Salad	I serving	190	7	33

SALADS & SALAD DRESSINGS
	AMOUNT	CALORIES	FAT-GRAMS	% FAT
Antipasto w/ Low-Cal Dressing	I serving	170	9	48
Greek, Small	I	85	5	53
w/ Low-Cal Dressing	I	140	8	51
Tossed, Small	I	40	I	24
w/ Low-Cal Dressing	I	80	2	23

SANDWICHES
	AMOUNT	CALORIES	FAT-GRAMS	% FAT
Ham & Cheese	I	520	21	36
Submarine	I	590	28	43
Tuna Melt	I	700	37	48
Turkey	I	450	17	34
Vegetarian	I	620	30	44

LONG JOHN SILVER'S

CHICKEN
	AMOUNT	CALORIES	FAT-GRAMS	% FAT
Baked, Light Herb	I serving	120	4	30
Flavorbaked	I serving	110	3	27

	AMOUNT	CALORIES	FAT-GRAMS	% FAT
Planks	1 pc	120	4	30
	2 pcs	240	12	45

CHICKEN ENTRÉE
Flavorbaked

	AMOUNT	CALORIES	FAT-GRAMS	% FAT
1 piece over Rice w/ Baked Potato & Green Beans	1 serving	450	8	15
1 piece over Rice w/ Side Salad	1 serving	275	7	23
Kid's Meal, 2 pieces w/ Fries, Hushpuppy	1 serving	560	29	47
Planks w/ Fries, Hushpuppies & Coleslaw				
2 pieces	1 serving	490	26	48
3 pieces	1 serving	890	44	44
4 pieces, no Hushpuppy	1 serving	940	44	42

COMBINATION ENTRÉE

	AMOUNT	CALORIES	FAT-GRAMS	% FAT
Fish, Scallops w/ Fries, 2 Hushpuppies & Coleslaw	1 serving	970	46	43
Fish, Shrimp & Chicken w/ Fries, Hushpuppies & Coleslaw	1 serving	1,160	65	50
Fish, Shrimp & Clams w/ Fries, Hushpuppies & Coleslaw	1 serving	1,240	70	51

	AMOUNT	CALORIES	FAT-GRAMS	% FAT
Fish & Chicken w/ Fries, Hushpuppies & Coleslaw	1 serving	950	49	46
Fish & Chicken w/ Fries	1 serving	550	32	52
Fish & Chicken Kid's Meal w/ Fries, Hushpuppies & Coleslaw	1 serving	620	34	49
Fish & Shrimp w/ Fries, Hushpuppies & Coleslaw	1 serving	1,140	65	51
Flavorbaked Fish & Chicken (1 piece each) over Rice w/ Baked Potato & Green Beans	1 serving	540	10	17

DESSERTS

	AMOUNT	CALORIES	FAT-GRAMS	% FAT
Cheesecake, Pineapple Cream	1 serving	310	18	52
Cookies				
Chocolate Chip	1	230	9	35
Oatmeal Raisin	1	160	10	56
Pies				
Apple	1 serving	320	13	37
Cherry	1 serving	360	13	33
Lemon	1 serving	340	9	24
Pecan	1 serving	445	22	44
Pumpkin	1 serving	250	11	39
Walnut Brownie	1	440	22	45

	AMOUNT	CALORIES	FAT-GRAMS	% FAT
FISH & SHELLFISH				
Fish				
Baked, w/ Sauce	I serving	150	2	12
Batter-dipped	I pc	180	11	55
Catfish Fillet	I pc	205	12	53
Crispy	I serving	150	8	48
Flavorbaked	I serving	90	3	28
Kitchen Breaded	I serving	120	5	37
Lemon Crumb	3 pcs	150	1	6
Light Paprika	3 pcs	120	1	6
Scampi Sauce	3 pcs	170	5	26
SHELLFISH				
Clams, Breaded	I serving	525	31	53
Oysters, Breaded	I serving	180	9	45
Scallops, Battered	I serving	160	9	51
Shrimp				
Batter-dipped	I pc	30	2	60
Breaded	I serving	390	23	53
FISH & SHELLFISH ENTRÉES				
Fish Entrées				
Baked, w/ Sauce, Coleslaw & Mixed Vegetables	I serving	390	19	44
Catfish Fillet w/ Fries, 2 Hushpuppies & Coleslaw	I serving	860	42	44

	AMOUNT	CALORIES	FAT-GRAMS	% FAT
Crispy Fish, 3 pieces, w/ Fries, Hushpuppies & Coleslaw	I serving	980	50	46
Fish				
3 pieces w/ Fries, 2 Hushpuppies & Coleslaw	I serving	960	44	41
3 pieces w/ Rice, Green Beans, Coleslaw & Roll	I serving	610	13	19
Fish & Fries				
Kids Meal, 1 piece w/ Fries & Hushpuppy	I serving	500	28	50
2 pieces w/ Fries	I serving	610	37	55
3 pieces w/ Fries & 2 Hushpuppies	I serving	810	38	42
Fish & More, 2 pieces w/ Fries, Hushpuppies & Coleslaw	I serving	890	48	49
Flavorbaked				
2 pieces over Rice w/ Baked Potato & Green Beans	I serving	520	10	17
2 pieces over Rice w/ Side Salad	I serving	345	9	24
Homestyle, 6 pieces w/ Fries, 2 Hushpuppies & Coleslaw	I serving	1,260	64	46

	AMOUNT	CALORIES	FAT-GRAMS	% FAT
Kitchen Breaded, w/ Fries, Hushpuppies & Coleslaw				
2 pieces	1 serving	820	46	51
3 pieces	1 serving	1,260	64	46
Light Lemon Crumb, 2 pieces w/ Rice, Salad	1 serving	290	5	16
Light Paprika, 2 pieces w/ Rice & Small Salad	1 serving	300	2	6
Shellfish Entrées				
Clams w/ Fries, Hushpuppies & Coleslaw	1 serving	990	52	47
Oysters, 6 pieces w/ Fries & Coleslaw	1 serving	790	45	51
Scallops w/ Fries & Coleslaw	1 serving	160	9	51
Shrimp Breaded, w/ Fries, Hushpuppies & Coleslaw	10 pcs	840	47	50
	21 pcs	1,070	51	43
w/ Scampi Sauce	1 serving	120	5	38

SALADS & SALAD DRESSINGS
Salads

	AMOUNT	CALORIES	FAT-GRAMS	% FAT
Garden, w/ Crackers	1 serving	170	9	48

	AMOUNT	CALORIES	FAT-GRAMS	% FAT
Ocean Chef,				
w/ Crackers	l serving	250	9	32
w/o Crackers or				
Dressing	l serving	110	1	8
Seafood	l scoop	210	5	21
w/ Crackers	l serving	270	7	23
Shrimp, w/ Crackers	l serving	185	3	15
Side, w/o Dressing	l serving	25	1	36
Salad Dressings				
(1.5 oz)				
Bleu Cheese	l serving	225	23	92
Italian, Reduced-Cal	l serving	20	1	45
Sea Salad	l serving	220	21	86
Thousand Island	l serving	225	22	88

SANDWICHES & WRAPS

Sandwiches

	AMOUNT	CALORIES	FAT-GRAMS	% FAT
Batter-Dipped				
Chicken	1	280	8	26
Batter-Dipped Fish	1	340	13	34
Flavorbaked Chicken	1	355	15	37
Flavorbaked Fish	1	385	19	45
Homestyle Fish	1	510	22	39
w/ Fries & Coleslaw	l serving	870	38	39

Wraps

	AMOUNT	CALORIES	FAT-GRAMS	% FAT
Blazin Cajun w/ Shrimp	1	1,420	72	46
Caesar w/ Chicken	1	1,250	65	47
Tangy Tartar w/ Fish	1	1,380	71	46

	AMOUNT	CALORIES	FAT-GRAMS	% FAT
OTHER ITEMS				
Baked Potato				
(no topping)	1	165	1	6
Breadstick, Fried	1	110	3	25
Green Beans	1 serving	35	1	14
Chowder				
Clam, w/ Cod	1 serving	140	6	39
Seafood, w/ Cod	1 serving	140	6	39
Cole Slaw	1 serving	140	6	39
French Fries	1 serving	220	10	41
Hushpuppy	1 piece	70	2	26
Mixed Vegetables	1 serving	60	2	30
Rice Pilaf	1 serving	140	3	18
Roll	1	110	1	7
Seafood Gumbo				
w/ Cod	1 serving	120	8	60
Sauce				
Honey Mustard	1 oz	55	0	0
Mayonnaise	.5 oz	100	10	100
Malt Vinegar	1 oz	0	0	0
Seafood	1 oz	35	0	0
Sweet and Sour	.5 oz	20	0	0
Tartar	1 oz	120	11	85

McDONALD'S

BREAKFAST

	AMOUNT	CALORIES	FAT-GRAMS	% FAT
Biscuit, w/ Spread	1	260	13	45
Breakfast Burrito	1	320	20	56
Breakfast Sandwiches				

	AMOUNT	CALORIES	FAT-GRAMS	% FAT
Biscuit w/				
Bacon, Egg & Cheese	1	440	26	53
Sausage	1	430	29	61
Sausage & Egg	1	510	35	62
Egg McMuffin	1	290	12	37
Sausage McMuffin	1	360	23	58
w/ Egg	1	440	28	57
Cereal				
Cheerios, w/o Milk	1 serving	70	1	13
Wheaties, w/o Milk	1 serving	80	1	5
Danish				
Apple	1	360	16	40
Cheese	1	410	22	48
Cinnamon Roll	1	400	20	45
Eggs, Scrambled	2	160	11	62
Hotcakes				
Plain	1 serving	310	7	20
w/ Margarine				
(2 pats) & Syrup	1 serving	580	16	24
Muffins				
Lowfat Apple Bran	1	300	3	9
English Muffin	1	140	2	13
w/ Margarine	1	170	4	21
Sausage	1 serving	170	16	85

CHEESEBURGERS & HAMBURGERS

Cheeseburgers

Arch Deluxe	1	550	31	51
Arch Deluxe w/ Bacon	1	590	34	52
Cheeseburger	1	320	13	37

	AMOUNT	CALORIES	FAT-GRAMS	% FAT
Quarter Pounder w/ Cheese	1	530	30	50
Hamburgers				
Big Mac	1	560	31	50
Hamburger	1	260	9	31
Quarter Pounder	1	420	21	45
CHICKEN				
Chicken McNuggets	4 pcs	190	11	52
	6 pcs	290	17	53
	9 pcs	430	26	54
DESSERTS				
Apple Pie	1 serving	260	13	45
Cookies				
Chocolate Chip	1	170	10	53
McDonaldland	1 package	180	5	25
Reduced-Fat Ice Cream				
Cone, Vanilla	1	150	5	30
Sundae				
Vanilla	1	165	1	5
Hot Caramel	1	360	10	25
Hot Fudge	1	340	12	32
Strawberry	1	290	7	22
Toppings				
Caramel	1 serving	140	2	12
Hot Fudge	1 serving	130	4	27
Strawberry	1 serving	70	0	0
Sundae Nuts	1 serving	40	4	79

	AMOUNT	CALORIES	FAT-GRAMS	% FAT
DRINKS & SHAKES				
Drinks				
Apple Juice	6 oz	80	0	0
Coca-Cola Classic				
Child	1	110	0	0
Small	1	150	0	0
Medium	1	210	0	0
Large	1	300	0	0
Diet Coke				
Child	1	0	0	0
Small	1	0	0	0
Medium	1	0	0	0
Large	1	0	0	0
Hi-C Orange Drink				
Child	1	120	0	0
Small	1	160	0	0
Medium	1	240	0	0
Large	1	350	0	0
Milk, 1%	8 oz	100	3	27
Orange Juice	6 oz	80	0	0
Sprite				
Child	1	110	0	0
Small	1	140	0	0
Medium	1	210	0	0
Large	1	300	0	0
SHAKES				
Chocolate, small	1	360	9	23
Strawberry	1	360	9	23
Vanilla	1	360	9	23

	AMOUNT	CALORIES	FAT-GRAMS	% FAT
POTATOES				
French Fries				
Small	1 serving	210	10	43
Large	1 serving	450	22	44
Super Size	1 serving	540	26	43
Hash Browns	1 serving	130	8	55
SALADS & SALAD DRESSINGS				
Salads				
Garden	1 serving	35	0	0
Grilled Chicken				
Deluxe	1 serving	120	2	15
Croutons	1 package	50	2	27
Salad Dressings				
Caesar	1 pkt	160	14	78
Fat-Free Herb				
Vinaigrette	1 pkt	50	0	0
Ranch	1 pkt	230	21	82
Red French,				
Reduced-Calorie	1 pkt	160	8	45
SANDWICHES				
Grilled Chicken				
Deluxe	1	440	20	41
Crispy Chicken				
Deluxe	1	500	25	45
Fish Fillet Deluxe	1	560	28	45

	AMOUNT	CALORIES	FAT-GRAMS	% FAT
OTHER ITEMS				
Sauces				
Barbecue	I serving	45	0	0
Honey	I serving	45	0	0
Honey Mustard	I serving	50	5	90
Hot Mustard	I serving	60	4	60
Sweet and Sour	I serving	50	0	0

PIZZA HUT

(Serving size based on 1 slice of medium pizza)

THIN 'N CRISPY				
Beef	I slice	230	11	43
Chunky Combo	I slice	250	13	47
Chunky Meat	I slice	295	17	52
Chunky Veggie	I slice	195	8	37
Cheese	I slice	225	10	40
Italian Sausage	I slice	280	17	32
Meat Lovers	I slice	300	16	48
Pepperoni Lovers	I slice	320	19	53
Pork	I slice	240	12	45
Supreme	I slice	260	14	28
Super Supreme	I slice	255	12	42
Veggie Lovers	I slice	190	8	38
HAND-TOSSED				
Beef	I slice	260	10	35
Cheese	I slice	255	9	32
Chunky Combo	I slice	280	15	48

	AMOUNT	CALORIES	FAT-GRAMS	% FAT
Chunky Meat	1 slice	325	16	44
Chunky Veggie	1 slice	225	6	24
Italian Sausage	1 slice	315	15	43
Meat Lovers	1 slice	320	15	42
Pepperoni Lovers	1 slice	335	16	43
Pork	1 slice	270	11	37
Supreme	1 slice	290	12	37
Super Supreme	1 slice	275	10	33
Veggie Lovers	1 slice	220	7	29
PAN PIZZA				
Beef	1 slice	290	18	56
Cheese	1 slice	280	13	42
Chunky Combo	1 slice	305	16	47
Chunky Meat	1 slice	350	20	51
Chunky Veggie	1 slice	250	10	40
Italian Sausage	1 slice	400	24	54
Meat Lovers	1 slice	350	23	59
Pepperoni Lovers	1 slice	360	25	63
Pork	1 slice	300	19	57
Supreme	1 slice	315	16	46
Super Supreme	1 slice	300	19	57
Veggie Lovers	1 slice	250	15	54
PERSONAL PAN, WHOLE				
Pepperoni	1	675	30	40
Supreme	1	650	35	48

	AMOUNT	CALORIES	FAT-GRAMS	% FAT
BIG FOOT				
Cheese	I slice	180	5	25
Pepperoni	I slice	195	7	32
Pepperoni, Mushroom & Sausage	I slice	215	9	38
STUFFED CRUST				
w/ Pepperoni & topped w/ Ham	I slice	440	17	34
TRIPLE DECKER				
w/ Ham	I slice	400	17	38

POPEYE'S

	AMOUNT	CALORIES	FAT-GRAMS	% FAT
CHICKEN				
Breast, Mild or Spicy	I serving	270	16	53
Leg, Mild or Spicy	I serving	120	7	55
Nuggets	I serving	410	32	70
Thigh, Mild or Spicy	I serving	300	23	68
Wing, Mild or Spicy	I serving	160	11	60
OTHER ITEMS				
Apple pie	I serving	290	16	49
Biscuit	I	250	15	54
Coleslaw	I serving	150	11	68
Corn on the Cob	I	90	3	29
French Fries	I serving	240	12	46
Onion Rings	I serving	310	19	56
Red Beans & Rice	I serving	270	17	56

RAX

	AMOUNT	CALORIES	FAT-GRAMS	% FAT
DESSERTS				
Chocolate Chip				
Cookie	1	130	6	42
Pudding				
Butterscotch	1 serving	140	6	39
Chocolate	1 serving	140	6	39
Vanilla	1 serving	140	6	39
MILK SHAKES, W/WHIPPED TOPPING				
Chocolate	1	560	13	21
Strawberry	1	560	13	21
Vanilla	1	500	14	25
PASTA & SAUCE				
Pasta				
Pasta Shells	1 serving	170	4	21
Pasta/Vegetable				
Blend	1 serving	100	4	36
Rainbow				
Rotini	1 serving	180	4	20
Spaghetti	1 serving	140	4	26
Sauce				
Alfredo	1 serving	80	3	34
Mushroom	1 oz	15	0	0
Spaghetti	1 serving	80	0	0
w/ Meat	1 serving	150	8	48
Spicy Meat	1 serving	80	4	45

	AMOUNT	CALORIES	FAT-GRAMS	% FAT
POTATOES				
Baked				
Barbecue	I serving	730	24	30
Chili	I serving	700	23	30
Plain	I serving	270	0	0
w/ Margarine	I serving	370	II	27
w/ Sour Cream	I serving	400	II	25
w/ Cheese & Bacon	I serving	780	28	32
w/ Cheese & Broccoli	I serving	760	26	31
French Fries				
Regular	I serving	260	13	45
Large	I serving	390	20	46
SALADS & SALAD DRESSINGS				
Salads				
Chef's, w/o Dressing	I serving	230	14	55
Garden, w/o Dressing	I serving	160	II	62
Garden Gourmet,				
w/ Lite Dressing	I serving	135	6	40
Macaroni	½ cup	160	7	39
Pasta	½ cup	80	I	II
Potato	I cup	160	7	24
Three-Bean	½ cup	100	0	0
Salad Dressings				
Bleu Cheese	I tbsp	50	5	90
Lite	I tbsp	35	3	77
French	I tbsp	60	4	60
Italian	I tbsp	50	4	72
Lite	I tbsp	30	3	90

	AMOUNT	CALORIES	FAT-GRAMS	% FAT
Oil	1 tbsp	130	14	97
Poppy Seed	1 tbsp	60	4	60
Ranch	1 tbsp	45	5	100
Thousand Island	1 tbsp	70	6	77
Lite	1 tbsp	40	3	68
Vinegar	1 tbsp	0	0	0

SANDWICHES

Beef				
Barbecue	1	420	14	30
Philly Beef				
& Cheese	1	480	22	41
Fish	1	460	17	33
Ham & Cheese	1	430	23	48
Roast Beef				
Small	1	260	14	48
Regular	1	320	11	31
Large	1	570	35	55
Turkey Club	1	670	43	58

OTHER ITEMS

Applesauce	1 cup	100	0	0
Barbecue Meat				
Topping	1 cup	140	4	26
Breadstick	1 oz	150	10	60
Cheese				
Cheddar, Tidbits	1 oz	160	11	62
Imitation,				
Shredded	1 oz	90	6	60

	AMOUNT	CALORIES	FAT-GRAMS	% FAT
Cheese Sauce				
Nacho	I cup	470	22	42
Regular	I cup	420	17	36
Chicken Noodle Soup	I cup	40	0	0
Coleslaw	I serving	70	4	51
Cottage Cheese	I cup	250	10	36
Hot Chocolate	6 oz	110	11	90
Refried Beans	I serving	120	4	30
Rice, Spanish	I serving	90	0	0
Sour Cream,				
Imitation	I cup	130	11	76
Taco Shell	I	40	2	45
Tortilla Chips	I oz	140	7	45

RED LOBSTER

DINNER PORTION

	AMOUNT	CALORIES	FAT-GRAMS	% FAT
Atlantic Cod, Fillet	I serving	200	2	9
Calamari Breaded,				
Fried	I serving	720	42	53
Catfish	I serving	340	20	53
Cherrystone Clams	I serving	260	4	14
Crab Legs				
King	I serving	170	2	11
Snow	I serving	150	2	12
Flounder	I serving	200	2	9
Grouper	I serving	220	2	8
Haddock	I serving	220	2	8
Halibut	I serving	220	2	8
Langostino	I serving	240	2	8

	AMOUNT	CALORIES	FAT-GRAMS	% FAT
Lobster				
Maine	l serving	240	8	30
Rock	l serving	230	3	12
Mackerel	l serving	380	24	57
Monkfish	l serving	220	2	8
Ocean Perch	l serving	260	8	28
Pollock	l serving	240	2	8
Red Rockfish	l serving	180	2	10
Red Snapper	l serving	220	2	8
Salmon				
Norwegian	l serving	460	24	47
Sockeye	l serving	320	8	23
Scallops				
Calico	l serving	360	4	10
Deep Sea	l serving	260	4	14
Shark				
Blacktip	l serving	300	2	6
Mako	l serving	280	2	6
Sole, Lemon	l serving	200	8	36
Tilefish	l serving	200	4	18
Trout, Rainbow	l serving	340	18	48
Tuna, Yellowfin	l serving	360	12	30

LUNCH PORTION

	AMOUNT	CALORIES	FAT-GRAMS	% FAT
Atlantic Cod, Fillet	l serving	100	1	9
Calamari Breaded, Fried	l serving	360	21	53
Catfish	l serving	170	10	53
Cherrystone Clams	l serving	130	2	14

	AMOUNT	CALORIES	FAT-GRAMS	% FAT
Flounder	1 serving	100	1	9
Grouper	1 serving	110	1	8
Haddock	1 serving	110	1	8
Halibut	1 serving	110	1	8
Langostino	1 serving	120	1	8
Mackerel	1 serving	190	12	57
Monkfish	1 serving	110	1	8
Ocean Perch	1 serving	130	4	28
Pollock	1 serving	120	1	8
Red Rockfish	1 serving	90	1	10
Red Snapper	1 serving	110	1	8
Salmon				
Norwegian	1 serving	230	12	47
Sockeye	1 serving	160	4	23
Scallops				
Calico	1 serving	180	2	10
Deep Sea	1 serving	130	2	14
Shark				
Blacktip	1 serving	150	1	6
Mako	1 serving	140	1	6
Sole, Lemon	1 serving	120	1	8
Swordfish	1 serving	100	4	36
Tilefish	1 serving	100	2	18
Trout, Rainbow	1 serving	170	9	48
Tuna, Yellowfin	1 serving	180	6	30
OTHER ITEMS				
Catfish, Breast	1 serving	120	3	23
Hamburger	1	320	23	65
Mussels	1 serving	70	2	26

	AMOUNT	CALORIES	FAT-GRAMS	% FAT
Oysters, Raw	6	110	4	33
Shrimp	8–10			
	pcs	120	2	15
Strip Steak	1 serving	690	64	83

SHAKEY'S PIZZA

(Serving size: ¹⁄₁₀ of 12" pie)

HOMESTYLE PAN CRUST

Cheese	1 slice	305	14	42
Pepperoni	1 slice	345	15	39
Sausage & Mushroom	1 slice	345	17	45
Onion, Green Peppers,				
Olives & Mushrooms	1 slice	320	15	42
Sausage & Pepperoni	1 slice	375	20	48
Shakey's Special	1 slice	385	21	49

THICK CRUST

Cheese	1 slice	170	5	27
Pepperoni	1 slice	185	6	29
Sausage & Mushroom	1 slice	180	6	30
Onion, Green Peppers,				
Olives & Mushrooms	1 slice	160	4	22
Sausage & Pepperoni	1 slice	180	8	41
Shakey's Special	1 slice	210	8	35

THIN CRUST

Cheese	1 slice	135	5	34
Pepperoni	1 slice	150	7	43

	AMOUNT	CALORIES	FAT-GRAMS	% FAT
Sausage & Mushroom	1 slice	140	6	38
Onion, Green Peppers,				
Olives & Mushrooms	1 slice	125	5	36
Sausage & Pepperoni	1 slice	165	8	43
Shakey's Special	1 slice	170	9	47
OTHER ITEMS				
Chicken, Fried				
w/ Potatoes	3 pcs	950	56	53
	5 pcs	1,700	90	48
Potato Wedges	15 pcs	950	36	34
Sandwich				
Ham & Cheese	1	550	21	34
Super Hot Hero	1	810	44	49
Spaghetti Entrée				
w/ Meat Sauce				
& Garlic Bread	1 serving	940	33	32

SHONEY'S

BREAKFAST

	AMOUNT	CALORIES	FAT-GRAMS	% FAT
Biscuit	1	170	8	43
Bacon	3 strips	110	9	78
Croissant	1	260	16	55
Egg, Fried	1	160	15	83
Grits	1 serving	60	3	51
Ham	2 slices	60	2	32
Honey Bun Pastry	1	265	14	48
Pancake	1	90	.5	5
Sausage	1 patty	105	10	84

	AMOUNT	CALORIES	FAT-GRAMS	% FAT
DESSERTS				
Apple Pie, à la Mode	1 serving	490	23	42
Brownie, à la Mode	1 serving	575	34	53
Carrot Cake	1 serving	500	26	47
Hot Fudge Cake	1 serving	525	20	34
Strawberry Pie	1 serving	330	17	45
CHEESEBURGERS &				
HAMBURGERS				
Cheeseburgers				
Hamburger Patty	1	290	23	71
Mushroom/Swiss	1	615	42	61
Patty Melt	1	640	42	59
Hamburgers				
All American	1	500	33	59
Old Fashioned	1	470	28	54
Shoney Burger	1	498	36	65
w/ Bacon	1	590	40	61
ENTRÉES				
Chicken				
Charbroiled, Lightside	1	240	7	26
Tenders, America's Favorites	1	390	20	47
Fish & Seafood				
Baked, Lightside	1 serving	170	1	5
Fried, Light	1 serving	300	14	44

	AMOUNT	CALORIES	FAT-GRAMS	% FAT
Fish & Chips	I serving	640	35	49
Fish 'N Shrimp	I serving	490	26	47
Seafood Platter	I serving	565	28	45
Shrimp				
Bite-size	I serving	390	25	57
Boiled	I serving	95	I	10
Charbroiled	I serving	140	3	20
Sampler	I serving	410	23	50
Shrimper's Feast	I serving	385	22	52
Large	I serving	575	33	52
Italian				
Italian Feast	I serving	500	20	35
Lasagna				
America's Favorites	I serving	300	10	30
Lightside	I serving	300	10	30
Spaghetti				
America's Favorites	I serving	495	16	30
Lightside	I serving	250	27	55
Liver & Onions	I serving	410	23	50
Steak				
Country Fried	I serving	450	27	55
Sirloin Steak	I serving	350	25	62
Steak 'N Shrimp				
Charbroiled	I serving	360	23	56
Fried	I serving	510	33	58
Rib Eye Steak				
& Chicken	I serving	605	51	75
Steak & Hawaiian				
Chicken	I serving	260	7	25
Steak & Chicken	I serving	240	7	28

SHONEY'S

	AMOUNT	CALORIES	FAT-GRAMS	% FAT
POTATOES				
Baked	1	265	0	0
French Fries				
Small	1 serving	190	8	36
Large	1 serving	250	10	35
Home Fries	1 serving	115	4	29
Hash Browns	1 serving	90	3	31
SALADS & SALAD DRESSINGS				
Salads				
Ambrosia	¼ cup	75	3	40
Apple Grape Surprise	¼ cup	20	0	0
Beet Onion	¼ cup	25	1	47
Broccoli Cauliflower	¼ cup	100	9	78
w/ Carrot	¼ cup	55	4	75
Carrot Apple	¼ cup	100	9	83
Coleslaw	¼ cup	70	5	67
Cucumber, Lite	¼ cup	10	0	0
Don's Pasta	¼ cup	80	5	50
Fruit Delight	¼ cup	55	2	27
Italian Vegetable	¼ cup	10	0	0
Kidney Bean	¼ cup	55	2	34
Macaroni	¼ cup	210	14	60
Mixed Fruit	¼ cup	40	0	0
Mixed Squash	¼ cup	50	4	75
Oriental	¼ cup	80	3	31
Pea	¼ cup	75	6	68
Rotelli Pasta	¼ cup	80	4	46
Saigon	¼ cup	70	4	51
Snow	¼ cup	70	4	51

	AMOUNT	CALORIES	FAT-GRAMS	% FAT
Spaghetti	¼ cup	80	5	51
Spring	¼ cup	40	3	69
Summer	¼ cup	115	12	92
Three Bean	¼ cup	95	5	48
Waldorf	¼ cup	80	5	58
Salad Dressings				
Biscayne, Low-Calorie	2 tbsp	60	1	15
Blue Cheese	2 tbsp	115	13	100
French	2 tbsp	125	12	87
Rue	2 tbsp	120	10	74
Honey Mustard	2 tbsp	165	17	93
Italian				
Creamy	2 tbsp	135	15	97
Golden	2 tbsp	140	15	96
Nonfat	2 tbsp	10	0	0
Ranch	2 tbsp	95	10	95
Thousand Island	2 tbsp	130	13	90
SANDWICHES				
Cheese				
Grilled	1	455	29	57
Grilled w/ Bacon	1	440	28	58
Chicken				
Charbroiled	1	450	17	34
Fillet	1	465	21	41
Fish	1	325	13	35
Ham				
Baked	1	290	10	32
Club	1	640	36	50

	AMOUNT	CALORIES	FAT-GRAMS	% FAT
Reuben	1	600	35	52
Slim Jim	1	485	24	44
Steak				
Country Fried	1	590	26	39
Philly	1	675	44	59
Turkey Club	1	635	33	46

SOUPS

	AMOUNT	CALORIES	FAT-GRAMS	% FAT
Bean	1 serving	65	1	16
Beef	1 serving	85	3	31
Broccoli, Cream of	1 serving	75	5	55
Cheese	1 serving	110	8	64
Broccoli-Cauliflower	1 serving	125	9	67
Chicken				
Cream of	1 serving	135	9	59
Gumbo	1 serving	60	2	30
Noodle	1 serving	60	1	20
Rice	1 serving	70	.5	6
Vegetable,				
Cream of	1 serving	80	1	15
Chowder				
Cheddar	1 serving	90	2	23
Clam	1 serving	95	5	52
Corn	1 serving	150	5	29
Onion	1 serving	30	2	62
Potato	1 serving	100	3	27
Tomato				
Florentine	1 serving	65	1	16
Vegetable	1 serving	45	.5	10
Vegetable Beef	1 serving	80	2	16

	AMOUNT	CALORIES	FAT-GRAMS	% FAT
OTHER ITEMS				
Barbecue Sauce	1 serving	40	1	22
Cocktail Sauce	1 serving	35	0	0
Country Gravy	3 oz	115	10	77
Mushrooms, Sautéed	1 serving	75	6	78
Onions, Sautéed	1 serving	40	2	51
Onion Ring	1	50	3	54
Rice	1 serving	140	4	24
Sundae				
Hot Fudge	1 serving	450	22	44
Strawberry	1 serving	380	19	45
Sweet & Sour Sauce	1 serving	60	0	0
Tartar Sauce	1 serving	85	8	83

SKIPPER'S

CHICKEN

	AMOUNT	CALORIES	FAT-GRAMS	% FAT
Lite Catch, 3 pieces, w/ Small Green Salad	1 serving	305	15	44
Strips				
Create A Catch	1 serving	80	4	44
Tenderloin Strips, 5 pieces, w/ Fries	1 serving	795	38	43

COMBINATION ENTRÉES

	AMOUNT	CALORIES	FAT-GRAMS	% FAT
Chicken Strips, 1 piece Fish & Fries	1 serving	805	40	45
Shrimp & Fries	1 serving	800	39	44

SKIPPE

	AMOUNT	CALORIES	FAT-GRAMS	% FAT
Clam Strips, 1 piece				
Fish & Fries	1 serving	870	54	56
Jumbo Shrimp,				
1 piece Fish & Fries	1 serving	720	36	45
Lite Catch, 1 piece Fish,				
2 pieces Chicken,				
Green Salad	1 serving	400	21	47
Shrimp, 1 piece Fish				
& Fries	1 serving	730	37	46
Oysters, 1 piece Fish				
& Fries	1 serving	885	44	45
FISH				
Clam Strips w/ Fries	1 serving	1,005	70	63
Cod, Thick cut				
3 pieces w/ Fries	1 serving	665	32	43
4 pieces w/ Fries	1 serving	760	36	43
5 pieces w/ Fries	1 serving	855	41	43
Fish Fillet	1 serving	175	10	51
1 piece w/ Fries	1 serving	560	28	45
2 pieces				
w/ Fries	1 serving	735	38	47
w/ Green Salad	1 serving	410	23	51
3 pieces w/ Fries	1 serving	910	48	48
Oyster Basket				
w/ Fries	1 serving	1,040	51	44
Salmon, Baked	1 serving	270	11	37
Seafood Entrée				
w/ Fries, Skipper's				
Platter Basket	1 serving	1,038	63	55

	AMOUNT	CALORIES	FAT-GRAMS	% FAT
Shrimp Basket				
Original w/ Fries	1 serving	725	36	45
Jumbo w/ Fries	1 serving	710	35	45
Shrimp w/ Seafood				
Sauce	1 serving	170	3	16

SALADS & SALAD DRESSINGS

Salads

	AMOUNT	CALORIES	FAT-GRAMS	% FAT
Green, Small	1 serving	60	3	46
Shrimp & Seafood	1 serving	170	3	16
Side	1 serving	25	0	0

Salad Dressings

	AMOUNT	CALORIES	FAT-GRAMS	% FAT
Blue Cheese	1 packet	220	23	93
Italian	1 packet	140	15	96
Low-Cal	1 packet	20	1	53
Ranch House	1 packet	190	20	96
Thousand Island	1 packet	160	14	79

SANDWICHES

	AMOUNT	CALORIES	FAT-GRAMS	% FAT
Chicken	1	605	32	48
Fish				
Create A Catch	1	525	33	57
Double	1	700	73	94

OTHER ITEMS

	AMOUNT	CALORIES	FAT-GRAMS	% FAT
Barbecue Sauce	1 tbsp	25	1	36
Chowder				
Alder Smoked				
Salmon	1 serving	165	7	38

	AMOUNT	CALORIES	FAT-GRAMS	% FAT
Clam, Create				
A Catch	1 cup	100	4	32
	1 pint	200	7	32
Cocktail Sauce	1 tbsp	20	0	0
Coleslaw	1 serving	290	27	84
French Fries	1 serving	385	18	42
Gelatin Dessert	1 serving	55	0	0
Milk, Low-fat	12 oz	180	10	50
Potato, Baked	1 serving	145	0	0
Root Beer Float	1 serving	300	10	30
Tartar Sauce	1 tbsp	65	7	97

SUBWAY

COOKIES

Chocolate Chunk	1	210	10	43
Chocolate Chip	1	210	10	43
Chocolate Chip				
M&M	1	210	10	43
Double Chocolate				
Brazil Nut	1	230	12	47
Oatmeal Raisin	1	200	8	36
Peanut Butter	1	220	12	49
Sugar	1	230	12	47
White Chocolate				
Macadamia Nut	1	230	12	47

DRINKS

Pepsi	12 oz	160	0	0
Diet Pepsi	12 oz	10	0	0

	AMOUNT	CALORIES	FAT-GRAMS	% FAT
Slice, Lemon-Lime	12 oz	150	0	0
Slice, Mandarin Orange	12 oz	170	0	0
Mountain Dew	12 oz	170	0	0

SALADS & SALAD DRESSINGS

Salads

	AMOUNT	CALORIES	FAT-GRAMS	% FAT
BLT	1 serving	140	8	51
Bread Bowl	1 serving	330	4	11
Chicken Taco	1 serving	250	14	50
Classic Italian BMT	1 serving	275	20	65
Club	1 serving	125	3	22
Cold Cut Trio	1 serving	190	11	52
Ham	1 serving	115	3	23
Meatball	1 serving	235	14	54
Pizza	1 serving	280	20	64
Roast Beef	1 serving	115	3	23
Roasted Chicken Breast	1 serving	160	4	23
Seafood & Crab	1 serving	245	17	62
Seafood & Crab w/ Light Mayo	1 serving	160	8	45
Steak & Cheese	1 serving	210	8	34
Subway Melt	1 serving	195	10	46
Tuna	1 serving	355	30	76
Tuna w/ Light Mayo	1 serving	205	13	57
Turkey Breast	1 serving	100	2	18
Turkey Breast & Ham	1 serving	110	3	25
Veggie Delight	1 serving	50	1	18

	AMOUNT	CALORIES	FAT-GRAMS	% FAT
Salad Dressings				
Creamy Italian	1 pkt	260	24	83
Fat-Free Italian	1 pkt	20	0	0
French	1 pkt	260	20	69
Fat-Free French	1 pkt	60	0	0
Thousand Island	1 pkt	260	24	83
Ranch	1 pkt	350	36	93
Fat-Free Ranch	1 pkt	50	0	0

SANDWICHES
(Nutritional values do not include cheese or condiments unless indicated.)

6" Cold Subs				
BLT	1	330	10	27
Classic Italian BMT	1	460	22	43
Club	1	310	5	15
Cold Cut Trio	1	380	13	31
Ham	1	300	5	15
Tuna	1	540	32	53
Tuna w/ Light Mayo	1	390	15	35
Turkey Breast	1	290	4	12
Turkey Breast & Ham	1	295	5	15
Roast Beef	1	305	5	15
Seafood & Crab	1	430	19	40
Seafood & Crab w/ Light Mayo	1	350	10	26
Veggie Delight	1	240	3	11

	AMOUNT	CALORIES	FAT-GRAMS	% FAT
6" Hot Subs				
Chicken Taco Sub	1	435	16	33
Roasted Chicken				
Breast	1	350	6	15
Steak & Cheese	1	400	10	23
Subway Melt	1	380	12	28
Meatball	1	420	16	34
Pizza Sub	1	465	22	43
Deli-Style				
Sandwiches				
Bologna	1	290	12	37
Ham	1	235	4	15
Roast Beef	1	245	4	15
Tuna	1	355	18	46
Tuna w/ Light				
Mayo	1	280	9	29
Condiments				
& Extras				
Bacon	2 slices	45	3	60
Cheese	2			
	triangles	40	3	68
Mayonnaise	1 tsp	40	4	90
Mayonnaise,				
Light	1 tsp	20	2	90
Mustard	2 tsp	10	0	0
Olive Oil Blend	1 tsp	45	5	100
Vinegar	1 tsp	0	0	0

SUBWAY

	AMOUNT	CALORIES	FAT-GRAMS	% FAT
TACO BELL				
BURRITOS				
Bean	1	390	12	28
Light	1	330	6	16
Beef	1	430	19	40
Big Beef Supreme	1	525	25	43
Light 7 Layer	1	440	9	18
Light Chicken	1	290	6	19
Light Chicken Supreme	1	410	10	22
Chili Cheese	1	390	18	42
Combo	1	410	16	35
Steak Supreme	1	500	23	41
Supreme	1	440	19	39
Light	1	350	8	21
SALADS & SALAD DRESSING				
Salads				
Seafood				
w/ Shell & Dressing	1 serving	860	55	58
Light				
w/ Chips	1 serving	680	25	33
w/o Chips	1 serving	330	9	25
w/ Shell, w/o Dressing	1 serving	650	42	58
w/o Shell & Dressing	1 serving	220	11	46
Taco				
w/ Shell & Dressing	1 serving	1,170	87	67

	AMOUNT	CALORIES	FAT-GRAMS	% FAT
w/ Shell,				
w/o Beans	l serving	820	57	62
w/ Shell	l serving	485	31	58
Light				
w/ Chips	l serving	680	25	33
w/o Chips	l serving	330	9	25
Salad Dressing				
Ranch	l pkt	235	25	95
TACOS & TOSTADAS				
Tacos				
Bellgrande	l	335	23	62
Chicken Soft	l	225	10	40
Light	l	180	5	25
Fajita	l serving	235	11	42
Light	l	140	5	32
Soft	l	180	5	25
Light Supreme	l	160	5	28
Soft	l	200	5	23
Platter, Light	l serving	1,060	58	49
Regular	l	180	11	55
Soft	l	220	11	45
Steak, Soft	l	220	9	37
Supreme	l	230	15	59
Soft	l	270	16	53
Tostadas				
Beef	l	240	11	41
Chicken	l	265	15	51

TACO BELL

	AMOUNT	CALORIES	FAT-GRAMS	% FAT
OTHER ITEMS				
Chicken Fajita	1 serving	225	10	40
Cinnamon Twists	1	170	8	42
Mexican Pizza	1	575	37	58
Meximelt				
Beef	1	265	15	51
Cheese	1	260	15	53
Nachos	1 serving	345	18	47
Bellgrande	1 serving	635	34	48
Supreme	1 serving	365	27	66
Pinto Beans w/ Cheese				
& Red Sauce	1 serving	190	9	43
Sauces				
Cheese, Nacho	2 oz	105	8	70
Green Sauce	1 oz	5	0	0
Guacamole	¾ oz	35	2	53
Picante	1 oz	5	0	0
Pico de Gallo	1 oz	10	0	0
Salsa	½ oz	20	0	0
Taco Sauce	1 pkt	5	0	0
Seasoned Rice	1 serving	110	3	25
Sour Cream	¾ oz	45	4	78

TACO TIME

BURRITOS				
Bean, Soft	1	550	21	35
w/o Cheese	1	460	14	27
Casita w/o Sour Cream				
or Cheese	1	430	17	36

	AMOUNT	CALORIES	FAT-GRAMS	% FAT
Combo, Soft	1	550	24	39
w/o Cheese	1	460	14	27
Meat, Soft, w/o Cheese	1	470	19	37
Veggie	1	535	20	34
w/o Sour Cream	1	500	17	30
w/o Sour Cream or Cheese	1	480	13	25

SALADS

	AMOUNT	CALORIES	FAT-GRAMS	% FAT
Chicken Taco				
w/o Dressing	1 serving	435	19	39
w/o Dressing or Cheese	1 serving	380	15	35
Side Order, w/o Dressing or Cheese	1 serving	300	13	39
Taco, w/o Dressing	1 serving	350	16	41
Veggie, w/o Dressing or Cheese	1 serving	300	13	39

TACOS & TOSTADAS

Tacos

	AMOUNT	CALORIES	FAT-GRAMS	% FAT
Chicken, Soft	1	390	12	28
w/o Cheese	1	335	8	21
Flour, Soft, w/o Cheese	1	330	12	33

Tostadas

	AMOUNT	CALORIES	FAT-GRAMS	% FAT
Meat, w/o Sour Cream or Cheese	1	410	17	37

TACO TIME

	AMOUNT	CALORIES	FAT-GRAMS	% FAT

OTHER ITEMS

	AMOUNT	CALORIES	FAT-GRAMS	% FAT
Cheeseburger, Taco, w/o Dressing or Cheese	1	400	13	29
Mexican Rice, Brown	1 serving	160	2	11
Refried Beans, w/o Cheese	1 serving	295	11	34
Sauce				
Casa	1 oz	40	0	0
Enchilada	1 oz	15	0	0
Hot	1 oz	10	0	0
Ranchero	2 oz	20	1	50

TCBY

REGULAR FROZEN YOGURT

	AMOUNT	CALORIES	FAT-GRAMS	% FAT
Kiddie	3.2 oz	105	2	17
Small	5.9 oz	190	4	19
Regular	8.2 oz	270	6	20
Large	10.5 oz	340	8	21
Super	15.2 oz	495	11	20
Giant	31.6 oz	1,030	24	21

NONFAT FROZEN YOGURT

	AMOUNT	CALORIES	FAT-GRAMS	% FAT
Kiddie	3.2 oz	90	0	0
Small	5.9 oz	160	0	0
Regular	8.2 oz	225	0	0
Large	10.5 oz	290	0	0
Super	15.2 oz	420	0	0
Giant	31.6 oz	870	0	0

	AMOUNT	CALORIES	FAT-GRAMS	% FAT
NONFAT, SUGAR-FREE				
FROZEN YOGURT				
Kiddie	3.2 oz	65	0	0
Small	5.9 oz	120	0	0
Regular	8.2 oz	165	0	0
Large	10.5 oz	210	0	0
Super	15.2 oz	305	0	0
Giant	31.6 oz	630	0	0

WENDY'S

	AMOUNT	CALORIES	FAT-GRAMS	% FAT
BREAKFAST				
Bacon	1 strip	30	2	60
Breakfast Sandwich	1	370	19	46
w/ Bacon	1	430	23	48
w/ Sausage	1	570	37	58
Biscuit	1	320	17	48
Danish				
Apple	1	360	14	35
Cheese	1	430	21	44
Cinnamon Raisin	1	430	21	44
Eggs, Scrambled	1 serving	190	12	57
French Toast	2 slices	400	19	43
Omelet				
Ham & Cheese	1 serving	290	21	65
Ham, Cheese & Mushroom	1 serving	290	21	65
Ham, Cheese, Onion & Green Pepper	1 serving	280	19	61

	AMOUNT	CALORIES	FAT-GRAMS	% FAT
Mushroom, Green Pepper & Onion	1 serving	210	15	64
Sausage	1 patty	200	18	81

CHEESEBURGERS & HAMBURGERS

Cheeseburgers

	AMOUNT	CALORIES	FAT-GRAMS	% FAT
Double	1	620	36	52
Jr.	1	320	13	37
Jr. Bacon	1	380	19	45
Jr. Deluxe	1	360	17	43
Kid's Meal	1	320	13	37
Single w/ Everything	1	420	20	43

Hamburgers

	AMOUNT	CALORIES	FAT-GRAMS	% FAT
Big Bacon Classic	1	580	30	47
Double	1	680	39	52
Jr.	1	270	10	33
Kid's Meal	1	270	10	33
Plain Single	1	360	16	40

CHICKEN

	AMOUNT	CALORIES	FAT-GRAMS	% FAT
Chicken Nuggets	5 pieces	210	14	60
Kids	4 pieces	170	11	58

CHILI

	AMOUNT	CALORIES	FAT-GRAMS	% FAT
Small	1 serving	210	7	30
Large	1 serving	310	10	29
Cheddar Cheese, Shredded	2 tsp	70	6	77

	AMOUNT	CALORIES	FAT-GRAMS	% FAT
DESSERTS				
Chocolate Chip Cookie	1	270	13	43
Frosty Dairy Dessert				
Small	1	330	8	22
Medium	1	440	11	23
Large	1	540	14	23
DRINKS				
Milk				
2%	8 oz	110	4	33
Chocolate	8 oz	160	5	28
Coca-Cola, Medium	1	150	0	0
Small	1	100	0	0
Large	1	200	0	0
Biggie	1	350	0	0
Diet Coke, Small	1	0	0	0
Dr Pepper, Small	1	100	0	0
Hot Chocolate	1	110	1	8
Lemonade	1	90	0	0
Lemon-Lime	1	100	0	0
Milk, 2%	1	110	4	33
POTATOES				
Baked				
Plain	1	310	0	0
Bacon & Cheese	1	530	18	31
Broccoli & Cheese	1	470	14	27
Cheese	1	570	23	36
Chili & Cheese	1	630	24	34
Sour Cream & Chives	1	380	6	14

	AMOUNT	CALORIES	FAT-GRAMS	% FAT
French Fries				
Small	1 serving	270	13	43
Medium	1 serving	390	19	44
Biggie	1 serving	470	23	44
Hash Browns	1 serving	360	22	55

SALADS & SALAD DRESSINGS

Fresh Salads to go
(without dressings)

	AMOUNT	CALORIES	FAT-GRAMS	% FAT
Caesar Side	1 serving	100	4	36
Deluxe Garden	1 serving	110	6	49
Grilled Chicken	1 serving	260	9	31
Side	1 serving	60	3	15
Taco	1 serving	380	19	45
Taco Chips	15	210	11	47

Salad Bar
(Average servings unless otherwise indicated)

	AMOUNT	CALORIES	FAT-GRAMS	% FAT
Alfalfa Sprouts	1 oz	10	0	0
Alfredo Sauce	1 oz	35	1	26
Apple Topping	1 serving	130	0	0
Bacon Bits, Imitation	1 serving	10	0	0
Bananas	1	25	0	0
Blueberries	1 tbsp	5	0	0
Blueberry Topping	1 serving	60	0	0
Breadstick	1	130	3	21
Broccoli, Raw	½ cup	10	0	0
Cabbage, Raw	¼ cup	5	0	0
Cantaloupe, Fresh	2 pcs	20	0	0

	AMOUNT	CALORIES	FAT-GRAMS	% FAT
Carrots, Raw	¼ cup	10	0	0
Cauliflower, Raw	½ cup	15	0	0
Celery, Raw	1 tbsp	0	0	0
Cheese				
American	1 oz	90	7	70
Cheddar, Shredded	1 oz	110	10	82
Cottage	½ cup	110	4	33
Imitation, Shredded	1 oz	90	6	60
Mozzarella	1 oz	90	7	70
Parmesan, Grated	1 oz	130	9	62
Provolone	1 oz	90	7	70
Swiss	1 oz	90	7	70
Cheese Sauce	¼ cup	25	1	36
Coleslaw				
California	2 tbsp	45	3	60
Regular	¼ cup	80	5	56
Chow Mein Noodles	½ oz	70	4	51
Corn Relish	¼ cup	35	0	0
Croutons	2 tbsp	25	1	36
Cucumbers, Raw	3 slices	5	0	0
Fettuccine	2 oz	190	3	14
Flour Tortilla	1	110	3	25
Garbanzo Beans	1	45	1	20
Garlic Toast	1 pc	70	3	39
Grapes	¼ cup	30	0	0
Honey Sauce	½ oz	45	0	0
Honeydew Melon	2 pcs	20	0	0
Green Peppers, Fresh, ¼ cup	1	10	0	0
Lettuce	1 cup	10	0	0

	AMOUNT	CALORIES	FAT-GRAMS	% FAT
Margarine				
Liquid	½ oz	100	11	99
Whipped	1 tbsp	70	8	100
Mayonnaise	1 tbsp	90	10	100
Mushrooms, Raw	¼ cup	5	0	0
Mustard Sauce	1 oz	50	1	18
Onion, Raw	3 rings	0	0	0
Olives, Black	1	35	3	77
Oranges, Fresh, 2 oz	1	25	0	0
Pasta Medley, 2 oz	1	60	2	30
Pasta Salad, ¼ cup	1	35	0	0
Peaches, in Syrup,				
2 pcs	1	30	0	0
Pepperoni, Sliced	1 oz	140	12	77
Potato Salad, ¼ cup	1	125	11	79
Refried Beans	1	70	3	39
Rotini	1	90	2	20
Sauces				
Alfredo	2 tbsp	50	2	36
Cheese	2 tbsp	50	2	36
Picante	2 oz	20	0	0
Spaghetti	2 tbsp	40	0	0
Sour Cream	1	60	6	90
Sour Topping	1	60	5	78
Imitation, 1 oz	1	45	4	80
Spaghetti Sauce	1	30	0	0
w/ meat, 2 oz	1	60	2	30
Spanish Rice	1	70	1	13
Sunflower Seeds &				
Raisins, 1 oz	1	140	10	64

	AMOUNT	CALORIES	FAT-GRAMS	% FAT
Taco Chips, 2 oz	1	260	10	35
Taco Meat	1	110	7	57
Taco Shell	1	45	3	60
Tartar Sauce, 1 tbsp	1	120	14	100
Three Bean Salad, ¼ cup	1	60	0	0
Tuna Salad	1	100	6	54
Salad Dressings				
Blue Cheese	2 tbsp	180	19	95
French	2 tbsp	120	10	75
Fat-Free	2 tbsp	0	0	0
Italian Caesar	2 tbsp	150	16	96
Italian, Reduced-Calorie	2 tbsp	40	3	68
Hidden Valley Ranch	2 tbsp	100	10	99
Reduced-Calorie	2 tbsp	60	5	75
Salad Oil	1 tbsp	120	14	100
Thousand Island	2 tbsp	90	8	80
Wine Vinegar	1 tbsp	0	0	0
SANDWICHES, PITA (WITH DRESSING)				
Chicken Caesar	1	490	18	33
Classic Greek	1	440	20	41
Garden Ranch Chicken	1	480	18	34
Garden Veggie	1	400	17	38
Pita Dressings				
Caesar Vinaigrette	1 tbsp	70	7	90
Garden Ranch	1 tbsp	50	5	90

	AMOUNT	CALORIES	FAT-GRAMS	% FAT

WHATABURGER

BREAKFAST

	AMOUNT	CALORIES	FAT-GRAMS	% FAT
Bacon	1 slice	40	3	78
Biscuit	1	260	13	43
w/ Bacon	1	360	20	51
w/ Egg & Cheese	1	435	26	55
& Bacon	1	510	33	58
& Sausage	1	600	42	62
w/ Gravy	1	480	27	51
w/ Sausage	1	445	29	58
Breakfast Sandwich				
Breakfast on a Bun	1	520	34	59
Ranchero	1	530	35	59
w/ Bacon	1	365	19	48
Egg Omelet	1	290	13	40
Ranchero	1	320	16	45
Danish, Pecan	1	270	16	53
Eggs, Scrambled	1 serving	190	15	71
Muffin, Blueberry	1	240	8	30
Pancakes	1 serving	260	6	20
w/ Sausage	1 serving	425	21	45
Platter				
w/ Bacon	1 serving	695	44	57
w/ Sausage	1 serving	785	53	60
Sausage	1 serving	210	19	82

CHEESEBURGERS & HAMBURGERS

Cheeseburgers

	AMOUNT	CALORIES	FAT-GRAMS	% FAT
Double Meat	1	895	49	49
Jr. Burger	1	350	18	46

	AMOUNT	CALORIES	FAT-GRAMS	% FAT
Justaburger	1	310	16	46
Regular	1	670	33	44
Hamburgers				
Double Meat	1	825	42	46
Justaburger	1	265	12	39
Regular	¼ lb	225	17	68
	⅒ lb	90	6	60
Whataburger	1	600	26	39
DESSERTS				
Apple Pie	1 serving	235	12	46
Apple Turnover	1	215	11	45
Cookies				
Chocolate Chunk	1	250	16	58
Macadamia Nut	1	270	16	54
Oatmeal Raisin	1	220	7	28
Peanut Butter	1	260	14	46
DRINKS & SHAKES				
Drinks				
Iced Tea, Medium	1	5	0	0
Milk, 2%	1 serving	115	4	32
Orange Juice	6 oz	80	0	0
Soft Drinks, Medium				
Cherry Coke	1	150	0	0
Coca-Cola Classic	1	140	0	0
Diet Coke	1	0	0	0

	AMOUNT	CALORIES	FAT-GRAMS	% FAT
Dr Pepper	1	140	0	0
Root Beer	1	160	0	0
Sprite	1	140	0	0
Shakes				
Chocolate, Small	1	335	8	23
Strawberry, Small	1	320	8	22
Vanilla,				
Small	1	320	9	25
Medium	1	440	13	27
Large	1	660	19	26
Extra Large	1	880	26	27

ONIONS & POTATOES
Onions

	AMOUNT	CALORIES	FAT-GRAMS	% FAT
Onion Rings				
Regular	1 serving	225	13	52
Large	1 serving	495	29	52
Potatoes				
Baked, Plain	1	310	0	0
Topped w/				
Broccoli & Cheese	1 serving	455	10	20
Cheese	1 serving	510	16	29
Mushrooms	1 serving	360	2	4
French Fries				
Junior	1 serving	220	12	49
Large	1 serving	440	24	49
Regular	1 serving	330	18	49
Hash Browns	1 serving	150	9	54

	AMOUNT	CALORIES	FAT-GRAMS	% FAT
SANDWICHES				
Chicken				
Grilled	1	440	14	29
w/o Salad Dressing	1	385	9	21
Whatachick'n Deluxe	1	575	27	42
Fish				
Whatacatch	1	475	27	51
w/ Cheese	1	520	32	55
Steak	1	390	12	28
Turkey, Grilled	1	440	15	31
SALADS & SALAD DRESSINGS				
Salads				
Chicken, Grilled	1 serving	150	1	6
Garden	1 serving	55	.5	8
Salad Dressings				
French	1 pkt	250	20	72
Ranch	1 pkt	365	38	94
Thousand Island	1 pkt	260	27	86
Vinaigrette,				
Lite	1 pkt	35	2	50
TACOS & TAQUITOS				
Tacos				
Beef	1	325	12	33
Chicken	1	272	7	22
Taquitos				
Regular	1	310	19	55

	AMOUNT	CALORIES	FAT-GRAMS	% FAT
w/ Cheese	1	360	23	56
& Ranchero	1	370	23	56
Bacon	1	335	16	43
Potato	1	445	22	44
Ranchero	1	320	18	51
Sausage	1	445	26	53

WHITE CASTLE

BURGERS

	AMOUNT	CALORIES	FAT-GRAMS	% FAT
Cheeseburger	1	200	11	50
Hamburger	1	160	8	45

BREAKFAST
Breakfast Sandwich

	AMOUNT	CALORIES	FAT-GRAMS	% FAT
Sausage	1	195	12	55
Sausage & Egg	1	320	22	61

CHICKEN & FISH

	AMOUNT	CALORIES	FAT-GRAMS	% FAT
Chicken Sandwich	1	185	7	34
Fish Sandwich	1	155	5	29
w/ 1 tbsp Tartar Sauce	1	230	12	47

ONIONS

	AMOUNT	CALORIES	FAT-GRAMS	% FAT
Rings, Regular	1 serving	245	13	48

POTATOES

	AMOUNT	CALORIES	FAT-GRAMS	% FAT
Chips	1 serving	330	17	47
French Fries	1 serving	300	15	45

GENERIC FAST FOODS

BREAKFAST

	AMOUNT	CALORIES	FAT-GRAMS	% FAT
Biscuit	1	275	13	42
Croissant				
w/ Egg & Cheese	1	370	25	60
& Bacon	1	415	28	62
& Ham	1	475	34	64
& Sausage	1	525	38	65
Danish				
Cheese	1	355	25	63
Cinnamon	1	350	17	43
Fruit	1	335	16	43
English Muffin				
w/ Butter	1	190	6	27
w/ Cheese & Sausage	1	395	24	56
w/ Egg, Cheese				
& Canadian Bacon	1	385	20	47
& Sausage	1	490	31	57
French Toast				
w/ Butter	2 slices	360	19	47
Sticks	5	480	29	55
Hash Brown Potatoes	½ cup	150	9	54
Omelet, Ham &				
Cheese, 2 eggs	1 serving	255	18	62
Pancakes w/				
Butter &				
Syrup	3	520	14	24
Sausage	1 patty	100	8	72
Scrambled Eggs	2	200	15	68

	AMOUNT	CALORIES	FAT GRAMS	% FAT

CHICKEN

Breaded & Fried

	AMOUNT	CALORIES	FAT GRAMS	% FAT
Dark Meat	2 pcs	430	27	56
Wing & Breast	2 pcs	495	30	54
Fillet w/o Mayo	1 serving	515	29	51
w/ Cheese	1 serving	630	39	55
Nuggets, Plain	1 pc	50	3	54
	6 pcs	290	18	55
w/ Barbecue Sauce	6 pcs	330	18	49
w/ Honey	6 pcs	330	18	48
w/ Mustard Sauce	6 pcs	325	19	53
w/ Sweet & Sour Sauce	6 pcs	345	19	47

DESSERTS

	AMOUNT	CALORIES	FAT GRAMS	% FAT
Brownie	1	245	10	37
Fried Pie	1	265	14	47
Ice Cream Cone				
Small	1	110	3	25
Medium	1	230	7	27
Large	1	340	10	27
Ice Cream Cone, Dipped in Chocolate				
Small	1	150	7	42
Medium	1	300	13	39
Large	1	450	20	40
Ice Cream Sandwich	1	140	4	26
Soft-Serve Ice Cream				
w/ Cone	1	165	6	33

	AMOUNT	CALORIES	FAT-GRAMS	% FAT
Sundae				
Caramel	1	305	9	27
Hot Fudge	1	285	9	27
Strawberry	1	270	8	26
FISH				
Clams, Breaded & Fried	¾ cup	450	26	52
Crab, Soft Shell, Fried	1	335	18	48
Crabcake				
Baked	1	90	1	10
Fried	1	290	19	58
Fish Fillet, Battered/				
Breaded, Fried	1	210	11	47
w/ Tartar Sauce & Cheese	1	525	29	49
Oysters, Battered/				
Breaded, Fried	6	370	18	44
Scallops, Breaded, Fried	6	385	19	44
Shrimp, Breaded, Fried	6–8	455	25	49

CHEESEBURGERS & HAMBURGERS

(w/o mayonnaise or mayonnaise-type dressing)

Cheeseburgers				
Double	1	545	28	46
Large	1	610	33	49
Regular	1	320	15	42
Hamburgers				
Double	1	460	22	43
Large	1	511	27	48
Regular	1	275	12	39

	AMOUNT	CALORIES	FAT-GRAMS	% FAT
HOT DOGS				
Regular	1	240	15	54
w/ Chili	1	325	18	49
Corn Dog	1	460	19	37
MEXICAN FOOD				
Burritos				
Bean	2	450	14	27
Bean & Cheese	2	380	12	28
Bean & Chili Peppers	2	415	15	32
Bean & Meat	2	510	18	32
Bean, Cheese & Beef	2	330	13	35
Beef	2	525	21	36
Beef & Chili Peppers	2	425	16	35
Beef, Cheese & Red Chili Peppers	2	635	25	35
Chili Con Carne	1 cup	255	8	28
Chimichanga				
Beef	1	425	20	42
Beef & Cheese	1	445	24	48
Beef, Cheese & Red Chili Peppers	1	360	18	43
Enchilada				
Cheese & Beef	1	325	18	49
Cheese & Sour Cream	1	320	19	53
Cheese, Beef & Bean	1	345	16	42
Frijoles w/ Cheese	1 cup	225	8	31
Nachos				
Cheese	6–8	345	19	49

	AMOUNT	CALORIES	FAT-GRAMS	% FAT
Cheese & Jalapeño				
Peppers	6–8	610	34	50
Cheese, Beef,				
Beans & Jalapeño				
Peppers	6–8	570	30	49
Taco				
Small	1 serving	370	21	51
Large	1 serving	570	32	51
Taco Salad				
w/ Chili Con Carne	1.5 cups	290	13	41
w/ Beef & Cheese	1.5 cups	280	15	47
Tostada				
Bean & Cheese	1	225	10	40
Bean, Beef &				
Cheese	1	335	17	46
Beef & Cheese	1	315	16	46
Beef, cheese				
& Guacamole	2	360	23	58
PIZZA				
Cheese, 12"	1 pie	875	20	21
	⅛ pie	110	3	24
Meat & Vegetable,				
12"	1 pie	1,215	35	26
	⅛ pie	150	4	24
Pepperoni, 12"	1 pie	1,080	42	35
	⅛ pie	135	5	33
Supreme, 10"				
Thick & Chewy	½ pie	640	22	31
Thin & Crispy	½ pie	510	21	37

	AMOUNT	CALORIES	FAT-GRAMS	% FAT
ONIONS & POTATOES				
Onions				
Onion Rings	8–9	175	16	80
Potatoes				
Baked				
w/ Cheese	1	475	29	54
w/ Cheese & Bacon	1	450	26	52
w/ Cheese Sauce				
& Broccoli	1	400	21	47
& Chili	1	480	22	41
w/ Sour Cream				
& Chives	1	395	22	50
Chips	1 oz	150	10	60
French Fries				
Large	1 serving	360	19	47
Regular	1 serving	240	12	46
Mashed, w/ Whole				
Milk & Margarine	⅓ cup	65	1	14
SALADS & SALAD DRESSINGS				
Salads				
Chef	1.5 cups	270	16	54
Coleslaw	½ cup	90	8	80
Tossed, No Dressing	1.5 cups	30	0	0
w/ Cheese	1.5 cups	100	6	51
w/ Chicken	1.5 cups	105	2	17
w/ Pasta & Seafood	1.5 cups	380	21	49
w/ Shrimp	1.5 cups	110	2	16
Macaroni	½ cup	170	6	32

	AMOUNT	CALORIES	FAT-GRAMS	% FAT
Potato	½ cup	160	9	51
Waldorf	½ cup	90	5	50
Salad Dressings				
Blue Cheese	2 oz	340	34	90
French	2 oz	230	21	81
Italian	2 oz	325	34	94
Low-Calorie	2 oz	50	2	36
Oriental	2 oz	100	1	9
Thousand Island	2 oz	395	39	89
Wine Vinegar	2 oz	5	0	0

SANDWICHES
(Many typical deli sandiches are overstuffed.)

	AMOUNT	CALORIES	FAT-GRAMS	% FAT
Bacon, Lettuce & Tomato				
Deli	1	600	37	56
Regular	1	290	16	50
Bologna w/o Mayo	1	305	16	47
Cheese, Grilled	1	510	33	58
Chicken, Club	1	570	26	41
Chicken Salad				
Deli	1	535	32	54
w/ extra Mayo	1	655	46	63
Regular	1	255	20	71
Chicken, Sliced	1	310	15	44
Corned Beef w/o Mayo				
Deli	1	500	20	36
Overstuffed	1	760	37	44
Regular	1	295	10	30
Cream Cheese & Jelly	1	370	16	39

	AMOUNT	CALORIES	FAT-GRAMS	% FAT
Egg Salad				
Deli	1	545	31	51
w/ extra Mayo	1	665	44	60
Regular	1	285	13	41
Ham w/o Mayo				
Deli	1	565	27	43
w/ Mayo	1	665	40	54
Regular	1	285	16	51
w/ Cheese	1	390	24	55
Ham Salad	1	320	17	48
Liverwurst				
w/o Mayo	1	260	12	42
Peanut Butter	1	350	20	51
& Jelly	1	385	15	35
Reuben, Deli	1	920	50	49
Roast Beef w/o Mayo,				
Deli	1	565	4	38
Sirloin Steak (3 oz)	1	325	12	33
Submarine, 6–8"				
w/ Roast Beef				
& Mayo	1	410	13	28
w/ Salami, Ham				
& Cheese	1	455	19	37
Tuna Salad				
Deli	1	715	43	54
w/ extra Mayo	1	835	56	61
Deli, Overstuffed	1	860	50	53
w/ extra Mayo	1	975	63	59
Regular	1	585	28	43
Tuna	1	400	19	43